MANUAL of GYNECOLOGIC ONCOLOGY

MANUAL of GYNECOLOGIC ONCOLOGY

Enrique Hernandez, M.D., FACOG, FACS

Associate Professor and Director
Division of Gynecologic Oncology
The Medical College of Pennsylvania
Philadelphia, Pennsylvania

Neil B. Rosenshein, M.D., FACOG

Associate Professor of Gynecology and Obstetrics
Associate Professor of Oncology
The Johns Hopkins University School of Medicine
Associate Professor of Epidemiology
The Johns Hopkins University School of Hygiene
and Public Health
Baltimore, Maryland

Churchill Livingstone
New York, Edinburgh, London, Melbourne

Library of Congress Cataloging-in-Publication Data

Hernandez, Enrique.
  Manual of gynecologic oncology.

  Bibliography: p.
  Includes index.
  1. Generative organs, Female—Cancer—Handbooks,
manuals, etc. I. Rosenshein, Neil B. II. Title.
RC280.G5H47   1989   616.99′465   89-7367
ISBN 0-443-08642-7

Distributed in the United Kingdom by Churchill
Livingstone, Robert Stevenson House, 1–3 Baxter's
Place, Leith Walk, Edinburgh EH1 3AF, and by
associated companies, branches, and representatives
throughout the world.

Accurate indications, adverse reactions, and dosage
schedules for drugs are provided in this book, but it is
possible that they may change. The reader is urged to
review the package information data of the manufacturers
of the medications mentioned.

Production Designer: *Angela Cirnigliaro*
Production Supervisor: *Christina Hippeli*

Printed in the United States of America

First published in 1989

Preface

Our goal for the *Manual of Gynecologic Oncology* was for it to be compact and affordable. It is not intended to compete with the standard textbooks, but to be a handy pocket reference for physicians who treat women with gynecologic malignancies. The guidelines presented here are based on our experience and that of our mentors at The Johns Hopkins Hospital.

The manual contains twelve chapters and two appendices. Chapters 3, 4, and 5 are dedicated to each of the three most prevalent gynecologic malignancies: endometrial, cervical, and ovarian cancer. A brief summary of the clinical and epidemiologic features of each tumor is followed by a review of its histopathology. A detailed outline of the evaluation and management of patients with each of these malignancies is presented. Chapters 8, 9, and 10 are dedicated to three of the most common gynecologic oncology surgical procedures: radical hysterectomy, radical vulvectomy, and intracavitary irradiation; guidelines for the pre- and postoperative care of patients undergoing each of these procedures are described. Chapter 7, Chemotherapy, presents general guidelines, as well as a number of frequently used chemotherapy protocols. Since new protocols are constantly being developed and old ones frequently modified, the administration of chemotherapy should be under the supervision of a physician familiar with the drugs being used and the tumors being treated. The management of patients with cervical intraepithelial neoplasia and gestational trophoblastic neoplasia are described in Chapters 12 and 6, respectively. Nutritional support, blood component therapy, and the care of long-term venous catheters are covered in some detail in Chapters 1, 2, and 11; these topics are seldom covered in gynecology and gynecologic oncology textbooks.

A list of suggested readings follows each chapter. For in-depth coverage of the various gynecologic malignancies the reader is referred to these readings or to one of the many available standard textbooks (e.g., Gusberg, Shingleton, and Deppe's *Female Genital Cancer* and the third edition of Morrow and Townsend's *Synopsis of Gynecologic Oncology*).

Enrique Hernandez, M.D.
Neil B. Rosenshein, M.D.

Acknowledgments

We acknowledge the secretarial assistance of Mrs. Peggie Murphy, Mrs. Patricia Kelly-Byrne, and Ms. Fran Goldberg, and we are grateful to Ms. Donna Balopole and the staff of Churchill Livingstone. Finally, this manual would not have been possible without the constant support of our families in all our endeavors.

Contents

Appendix II

1

Nutritional Support of the Gynecologic Oncology Patient

Malnutrition is a frequent complication in the cancer patient. It can be secondary to the malignancy or to the therapy. Adequate nutrition is necessary for maintenance of body cell mass, metabolic processes, and tissue repair. Therefore, the gynecologic oncology patient should undergo periodic nutritional assessment and identification of any nutritional deficiencies that may need to be corrected.

NUTRITIONAL ASSESSMENT

SIMPLE MEASUREMENTS

The following simple measurements should be obtained from all gynecologic oncology patients.

Weight

Recent unintentional weight loss of 10% or greater may indicate malnutrition. Weighing less than 90% of ideal body weight may also indicate malnutrition.

Height

Height and frame size can be used to estimate the ideal body weight. An estimate of the female patient's ideal body weight can be obtained by allowing 100 pounds for the first 60 inches of height and adding 5 pounds for each additional inch. Subtract 10% for small frame. Add 10% for large frame. Frame size can be estimated by asking the patient to place her index finger and thumb around her wrist. If the thumb and index finger do not touch, she has a large frame. If they just touch, she has a medium frame. If they pass each other, she has a small frame.

Total Lymphocyte Count

A decrease in total lymphocyte count is seen with decreased visceral protein. A total lymphocyte count below 1,500/mm^3 may indicate malnutrition.

Serum Albumin

A serum albumin concentration of less than 3.5 g/dl may indicate malnutrition.

ADDITIONAL MEASUREMENTS

If any of the above criteria is present, further measurements will help clarify the patient's nutritional status.

Skin Tests

A negative response to skin testing, for example, *Candida*, mumps, streptodornase-streptokinase, and purified protein derivative (PPD), indicates depressed cellular immunity and indirectly visceral protein status.

Serum Transferrin

Serum transferrin has a half-life of 8 days compared with 19 days for serum albumin. Therefore, serum transferrin will show decreased levels sooner in the presence of decreased visceral protein.

Anthropometric Measurements

Muscle and fat wasting can be measured by the mid-arm muscle circumference and the triceps skinfold. These measurements are compared with that expected for age and sex and reported as percentage of normal.

DEFINITION OF MALNUTRITION

The severely malnourished woman will show obvious physical signs of protein malnutrition (kwashiorkor) or protein-calorie malnutrition (marasmus).

1. *Kwashiorkor:* The patient with severe protein malnutrition has changes in skin turgor, hair color, and consistency. There is edema, ascites, and enlargement of the liver and parotid gland.
2. *Marasmus:* The patient with severe protein-calorie malnutrition appears cachectic with muscle and fat wasting.

Most gynecologic oncology patients are not severely malnourished and do not present with obvious physical signs of malnutrition. Nevertheless, the patient should be strongly suspected of being malnourished if at least three of the following criteria are present:

1. Recent unintentional weight loss of 10% or greater
2. Total lymphocyte count below 1,500/mm^3
3. Serum albumin of less than 3.5 g/dl
4. Negative response to skin tests (anergy panel)
5. Serum transferrin of less than 200 mg/dl

DEGREE OF MALNUTRITION

An estimate of the degree of malnutrition can be obtained from the following table:

Test	Malnutrition		
	Mild	Moderate	Severe
Albumin (mg/dl)	3.0–3.5	2.5–2.9	<2.5
Transferrin (mg/dl)	180–200	160–179	<160
Lymphocytes (mm^3)	1,500–1,800	900–1,499	<900

NUTRITIONAL SUPPORT

Nutritional support of the malnourished patient is best accomplished via the gastrointestinal (GI) tract. If the GI tract cannot be used, peripheral parenteral nutrition (PPN) or total parenteral nutrition (TPN) through a central line should be considered as a viable option to provide caloric requirements and essential nutrients to promote anabolism.

CALORIC REQUIREMENTS

An average adult needs approximately 30 kcal/kg/day. This is a general guide. Other formulas are available, but they tend to overestimate. The above formula can be used and the caloric intake adjusted according to the patient's response.

To calculate the kilocalories (kcal) being delivered, the following formulas can be used:

kcal = grams of amino acids (protein) × 4
kcal = grams of carbohydrates × 3.4 (parenteral), or × 4 (enteral)
kcal = grams of fat × 9

The fat emulsion solutions (e.g., Intralipid 10%, Intralipid 20%) provide 1.1 or 2.0 kcal/ml of solution. The ratio of nonprotein calories to nitrogen should be 150–200:1. This may need to be lower (e.g., 100:1) in high-stress patients or higher (e.g., 300:1) in nitrogen-retaining states (e.g., acute renal failure, hepatic failure). It is recommended that no more than 60% of the total daily caloric intake be provided by fatty acids.

FLUID REQUIREMENTS

An average of 1,500 ml/m^2 of body surface area is needed per day. (The body surface area of a 66-inch tall, 140-pound woman is 1.5 m^2.) This woman will require 2,250 ml of fluids every 24 hours. The daily requirements for sodium and potassium are 60 mEq/m^2 and 30–40 mEq/m^2, respectively.

ENTERAL NUTRITION

The GI tract should be used whenever feasible. If the patient is eating, her diet can be supplemented with commercially available formulas. If the patient is not eating, tube feedings using a small-diameter (e.g., #8 Fr), soft, tungsten-tip feeding tube can be instituted. In surgical patients whose return of gastric or colonic function is expected to be delayed, administration of an elemental diet through a catheter jejunostomy should be considered. Elemental formulas (e.g., Vivonex, Vital High Nitrogen) are absorbed in the small intestine. Only 100 cm of small intestine is required for absorption.

Enteral Formulas

A large number of formulas are commercially available. It is best to be familiar with the generic features of the formulas and to select one or two products in each group for clinical use.

Intact Nutrient Formulas

Intact nutrient formulas are used in patients with normal GI tract function. These polymeric mixtures contain proteins, fats, and carbohydrates. They are almost isosmolar (approximately 350 mOsm/L) and supply 1 kcal/ml with approximately 30% of the calories being provided by fat. We prefer the lactose-free formulas (e.g., Enrich, Isocal, Precision Isotonic). Enrich, Isocal, and Precision are unpalatable and are recommended for tube feeding only. For oral feedings (diet supplementation), Ensure or Resource are recommended.

Predigested Nutrient Formulas

Predigested nutrient formulas have been labeled elemental because they use amino acids as the nitrogen source and oligosaccharides as the carbohydrate source. Most contain little fat and no lactose (e.g., Vivonex T.E.N., Vital High Nitrogen). They are helpful in patients who have an abnormal GI tract. They are the preferred formulas for infusion through a needle-catheter jejunostomy because of their low viscosity. They frequently cause diarrhea because of their high osmolality (550–850 mOsm/L). A new semielemental formula of low viscosity, Reabilan, has an osmolality of 350 mOsm/L. The above formulas supply 1 kcal/ml and a calorie-to-nitrogen ratio of 150–200:1. Special formulas for patients with renal failure (e.g., Travasorb Renal, Amin-Aid), chronic hepatic encephalopathy (e.g., Travasorb Hepatic, Hepatic-Aid) and for patients with respiratory insufficiency (Pulmocare) are available.

Tube Feedings

The continuous infusion is the simplest and safest way to administer tube feedings. It is the least time-consuming of all the tube-feeding techniques, resulting in maximum staff compliance. This method of nutrition allows for maximum control of the infusion rate and maximizes nutrient delivery. With the continuous infusion technique, there is the least chance for aspiration, nausea, gastric distention, cramping, and diarrhea. It requires a pump. This can result in limited ambulation if a battery-powered pump is not used. With this technique, the head of the bed needs to be elevated at least 30 degrees. A cyclic drip infusion can be used to allow the patient to have some time when she can be in bed without head elevation. Hyperosmolar medications (e.g., potassium chloride) should not be given through the tube, since they can cause diarrhea.

Infusion of enteral nutrient formulas through a nasogastric feeding tube is started at 50 ml/hr, using a lactose-free 1-kcal/ml formula, diluted to half-strength. Although intact nutrients formulas are almost isosmolar, some patients will develop diarrhea if the formula is started at full-strength. The half-strength dilution allows some time for GI adaptation to occur. On the second day, the infusion rate is increased to 100 ml/hr. If the half-strength formula is tolerated, a three-quarter strength formula is used on the third day, and a full-strength formula on the fourth day. When the patient is receiving the maximum tolerated concentration, the infusion rate is increased by 25 ml/hr every 8 hours until the desired rate is achieved.

Needle-Catheter Jejunostomy

Postoperative patients who receive a needle-catheter jejunostomy can start continuous infusion of a half-strength elemental formula in the recovery room at a rate of 50 ml/hr. On the second day of jejunostomy feeding, the rate is increased to 100 ml/hr. On the third day, the concentration of the formula is increased to three-quarters strength. If tolerated, it is increased to full-strength on the

TABLE 1-1. SUGGESTED FORMULATION
FOR PERIPHERAL PARENTERAL
NUTRITION

Component	Quantity
Dextrose 10%	500 ml
Travasol 5.5% with electrolytes	500 ml
Sodium	35 mEq/L
Chloride	35 mEq/L
Potassium	30 mEq/L
Phosphate	30 mEq/L
Magnesium	5 mEq/L
Acetate	50 mEq/L

fourth day. The infusion rate is then increased if necessary by 25 ml/hr every 24 hours, until the desired rate is achieved.

PERIPHERAL PARENTERAL NUTRITION

Peripheral parenteral nutrition can be used in patients needing nutritional support but who are not hypercatabolic and whose GI tract is expected to be functional within 5–7 days. It can also be used to supplement oral feedings in patients whose oral intake is inadequate.

Formula for Peripheral Parenteral Nutrition

A suggested formula for PPN is 500 ml Travasol 5.5% with electrolytes plus 500 ml 10% dextrose (Table 1-1). This will result in 1 L of solution containing 27.5 g of amino acids and 50 g of dextrose. It also contains 35 mEq/L of sodium and chloride, 30 mEq/L of potassium and phosphate, 5 mEq/L of magnesium, and 50 mEq/L of acetate. This solution has an osmolality of approximately 530 mOsm/L and contains 280 kcal/L. Infusing 2 L of this solution and 1 L of Intralipid 10% (1.1 kcal/ml) provides 1,660 kcal in 24 hours. Higher concentrations of dextrose (e.g., 10%) or amino acids (e.g., 4.25%) will universally cause phlebitis within 36–48 hours. The addition of 500 U of heparin and 5 mg of hydrocortisone sodium succinate (Solu-Cortef) to each liter of solution decreases

TABLE 1-2. MULTIVITAMINS

Vitamin	Quantity
M.V.I.-12 (to be added to 1 L/day)	
Vial 1	5 ml
Ascorbic acid (vitamin C)	100 mg
Retinol (vitamin A)	1 mg
Ergocalciferol (vitamin D)	5 μg
Thiamine (vitamin B_1)	3 mg
Riboflavin (vitamin B_2)	3.6 mg
Pyridoxine (vitamin B_6)	4 mg
Niacinamide	40 mg
Dexpanthenol	15 mg
Vitamin E	10 mg
Vial 2	5 ml
Biotin	60 μg
Folic acid	400 μg
Cyanocobalamin (vitamin B_{12})	5 μg

the risk of phlebitis. The simultaneous infusion of lipids and the hypertonic dextrose/amino acids solution through a Y-connector reduces the osmolality of the final infusate and reduces the incidence of phlebitis. The lack of a lipid free interval may promote intense hyperlipedemia.

Additional Additives

Multivitamins (e.g., M.V.I.-12) are added to one of the liters of parenteral nutrition solution once daily (Table 1-2). One ml of multiple trace metals is added to 1 L of solution every 24 hours (Table 1-3). Electrolytes can be supplemented as necessary by the addition of sodium chloride, sodium acetate, or sodium phosphate, potassium chloride, potassium acetate, or potassium phosphate, mag-

TABLE 1-3.   TRACE ELEMENTS

Elements	Quantity
Multitrace 5	1 ml
Zinc	1 mg
Copper	0.4 mg
Manganese	0.1 mg
Chromium	4.0 μg
Selenium	20 μg

nesium sulfate, and calcium gluconate. The chloride salts are used in the presence of metabolic alkalosis and the acetate salts in patients with metabolic acidosis.

Administration

Peripheral parenteral nutrition should be delivered through an infusion pump (e.g., IMED, IVAC). Parenteral nutrition solutions (dextrose/amino acids) should not hang for more than 24 hours. The fat emulsion solutions should not hang for more than 12 hours. The IV site used for parenteral nutrition should not be used for other purposes (e.g., antibiotics, chemotherapy). It should be routinely changed every 72 hours.

Severe allergy to eggs is a contraindication to the administration of fat emulsions (e.g., Intralipid). Lipid infusions can cause altered clotting function and decreased pulmonary function. The initial infusion rate should be 1 ml/min for the first 15 minutes. If no adverse reaction is observed, the infusion rate is increased to deliver 500 ml over 4 hours. Only 500 ml of fat emulsion is infused the first day. As a general rule, no more than 2.5 g of lipids per kg of body weight is given daily. The lipid infusion should provide no more than 60% of the total calories.

TOTAL PARENTERAL NUTRITION

Total parenteral nutrition provides enough calories to support a malnourished hypercatabolic patient with a defective GI tract. The osmolality of the total parenteral nutrition solutions is high (1,900 mOsm/L), necessitating a central venous line.

TABLE 1-4. SUGGESTED FORMULATION FOR
TOTAL PARENTERAL NUTRITION

Component	Quantity
Dextrose 25%	500 ml
Freamine III 8.5% with electrolytes	500 ml
Sodium	30 mEq/L
Chloride	30 mEq/L
Potassium	20 mEq/L
Magnesium	5 mEq/L
Calcium	5 mEq/L
Phosphate	10 mEq/L
Acetate	62 mEq/L

Add M.V.I.-12 (vial 1 and 2) to 1 L daily
Add 3 ml of Multitrace 5 to 1 L daily

Formula for Total Parenteral Nutrition

A mixture of 500 ml of Freamine III 8.5% plus 500 ml of 50% dextrose produces 1 L of solution containing 42 g of protein and 250 g of dextrose (Table 1-4). It provides 1020 kcal/L, with a non-protein calories to nitrogen ratio of 125:1. The amino acid solution (Freamine III 8.5%) with electrolytes contains 30 mEq/L of sodium and chloride, 20 mEq/L of potassium, 5 mEq/L of magnesium and calcium, 10 mEq/L of phosphate, and 62 mEq/L of acetate. A less hypertonic solution (e.g., 15% dextrose) may be used in patients who have poor glucose tolerance and in patients with compromised respiratory function in whom excessive carbon dioxide production can be a problem. In patients receiving long-term TPN, a 15% dextrose solution may prevent fatty infiltration of the liver. The infusion of 1 L of 15% dextrose/4.25% amino acids (1,400 mOsm/L) can be combined with 500 ml of fat emulsion (e.g., Intralipid 10%). This combination provides the same amount of calories and amino acids as the 25% dextrose/4.25% amino acid formula. The fat emulsion solutions have an osmolality of 280 mOsm/L and can be infused through a peripheral vein. These solutions supply 1.1 kcal/ml.

Additives

Multivitamins (Table 1-2) and trace elements (Table 1-3) are added to 1 L of hyperalimentation solution every 24 hours. The multivitamins include 3,300 IU of vitamin A, 200 IU of vitamin D, 10 IU of vitamin E, 100 mg of ascorbic acid, 3 mg of thiamine (B_1), 3.6 mg of riboflavin (B_2), 40 mg of niacin, 4 mg of vitamin B_6, 15 mg of pantothenic acid, 5 μg of vitamin B_{12}, 0.4 mg of folic acid, and 60 μg of biotin. The trace elements include 1.2 mg of copper, 3 mg of zinc, 12 μg of chromium, 60 μg of selenium, and 0.3 mg of manganese. In addition, 10 mg of vitamin K is given intramuscularly once a week, and 150 μg of vitamin B_{12} is given by IM injection once a month. Electrolytes can be supplemented as necessary (see the section *Nutritional Support, peripheral parenteral nutrition*). Additional potassium is usually necessary to bring the total potassium in each liter to 40–60 mEq. If no additional chloride is needed, the supplemental potassium can be given as potassium phosphate and/or potassium acetate.

Administration

Total parenteral nutrition solutions are hyperosmolar and require a central venous line for infusion. They should be delivered through an infusion pump. After placement of the central line and radiographic confirmation of its location in the superior vena cava, the patient is given 10% dextrose solution with electrolytes. After 24 hours on 10% dextrose, an infusion of 1 L of hyperalimentation solution (25% dextrose/4.25% amino acids) is started at 42 ml/hr (1 L in 24 hours). Additional fluid and electrolyte requirements are given through a peripheral line. If this is tolerated, 2 L of hyperalimentation solution is infused every 24 hours (84 ml/hr). This will provide the patient with 2,038 kcal/day. Additional calories can be provided by the use of fat emulsions (e.g., Intralipid 10%, 500–1000 ml/day). Fat emulsions should be given at least two to three times per week to provide essential fatty acids.

Severely malnourished patients tolerate the sudden increase in calorie intake poorly. In these patients, the hyperalimentation infusion should be progressively increased at a slow rate and under careful monitoring.

Complications

Hypoglycemia can occur as a result of a sudden discontinuation of hyperalimentation. This is usually related to mechanical problems with the central line. If this occurs, 10% dextrose is infused through a peripheral line at the same rate that the hyperalimentation solution was infusing.

Hyperosmolar hyperglycemic nonketotic coma can occur in patients with latent or unknown diabetes, pancreatitis, or sepsis, in patients on peritoneal dialysis, and in those receiving steroids or phenytoin. Careful monitoring of urine and blood glucose and administration of regular insulin as required to normalize blood glucose levels will prevent this complication.

Elevation of liver function tests usually occurs after 12–14 days on continuous hyperalimentation. Normalization occurs after hyperalimentation is discontinued. Excessive carbohydrate infusion can lead to increased synthesis of fatty acids and fatty infiltration of the liver. Therefore, this complication can be prevented by restricting the amount of carbohydrate calories (see the section *Nutritional Support, total parenteral nutrition*).

Hyperchloremic metabolic acidosis may occur because of the liberation of hydrochloric acid during the metabolism of amino acids. It is prevented by the addition of acetate to the hyperalimentation solution.

Dehydrated patients given a sudden large nitrogen load will develop prerenal azotemia. Adequate hydration before the initiation of hyperalimentation is therefore required.

The delivery of large amounts of carbohydrates results in increased production of carbon dioxide with a concomitant increase in minute ventilation. This could be disastrous in a patient with compromised pulmonary function. It can be avoided by the use of a less hypertonic solution (e.g., 15% dextrose).

Complications associated with the use of fat emulsions include hyperlipidemia, transient hypoxemia, microembolism, and elevated liver function test.

Other complications associated with TPN include acute acalculous cholecystitis, defective hemoglobin function, platelet dysfunction, refeeding anemia, and catheter-related complications.

MONITORING

When nutritional support seems indicated, a formal nutrition consult should be obtained. The following baseline studies should be ordered: height, weight, complete blood count (CBC), total lymphocyte count, serum electrolytes, calcium, magnesium, liver enzymes, prothrombin time (PT), partial thromboplastin time (PTT), serum albumin and transferrin, triglycerides, and 24-hour urine for urine urea nitrogen.

Nitrogen Balance

The nitrogen balance should be calculated twice a week (e.g., Tuesdays and Thursdays) if the patient has normal renal function. To calculate the nitrogen intake, the grams of protein supplied are divided by 6.25 (g nitrogen = g amino acids ÷ 6.25). The nitrogen balance can be calculated by the use of the following formula: nitrogen balance = nitrogen intake − (urine urea nitrogen + 3).

Follow-up Studies

The following studies are ordered for patients receiving nutritional support:

1. Daily weights
2. Fluid intake and output
3. Daily calorie count (nutrient intake analysis)
4. Urinalysis for glucose and acetone every 6–8 hours.
5. Weekly serum albumin, transferrin, PT, PTT, triglycerides
6. Twice a week (e.g., Tuesdays and Thursdays)
   a. CBC
   b. Total lymphocyte count
   c. Serum electrolytes, calcium, magnesium
   d. Liver enzymes

SUGGESTED READINGS

Abbott WC, Echenique MM, Bistrian BR, et al: Nutritional care of the trauma patient. Surg Gynecol Obstet 157:583, 1983
Bower RH, Talamini MA, Sax HC, et al: Postoperative enteral vs par-

enteral nutrition: A randomized controlled trial. Arch Surg 121:1040, 1986

Brennan MF: Total parenteral nutrition in the cancer patient. N Engl J Med 305:375, 1981

Craig RM, Neumann T, Jeejeebhoy KN, et al: Severe hepatocellular reaction resembling alcoholic hepatitis with cirrhosis after massive small-bowel resection and prolonged total parenteral nutrition. Gastroenterology 79:131, 1988

Dobbie RP, Hoffmeister JA: Continuous pump-tube enteric hyperalimentation. Surg Gynecol Obstet 143:273, 1976

Gazzaniga AB, Day AT, Sankary H: The efficacy of a 20 percent fat emulsion as a peripherally administered substrate. Surg Gynecol Obstet 160:387, 1985

Greenberg GR, Marliss EB, Anderson GH, et al: Protein-sparing therapy in post-operative patients: Effects of added hypocaloric glucose or lipid. N Engl J Med 294:1411, 1976

Hardin TC, Page CP, Schweisinger WH: Rapid replacement of serum albumin in patients receiving total parenteral nutrition. Surg Gynecol Obstet 163:359, 1986

Hoover HC, Ryan JA, Anderson EJ, et al: Nutritional benefits of immediate post-operative jejunal feeding of an elemental diet. Am J Surg 139:153, 1980

Irvin TT: Effects of malnutrition and hyperalimentation on wound healing. Surg Gynecol Obstet 146:33, 1978

Lindor KD, Fleming R, Abrams A, et al: Liver function values in adults receiving total parenteral nutrition. JAMA 241:2398, 1979

MacFayden BV Jr, Dudrick SJ, Ruberg RL: Management of gastrointestinal fistulas with parenteral hyperalimentation. Surgery 74:100, 1974

Michel L, Serrano A, Malt RA: Nutritional support of hospitalized patients. N Engl J Med 304:1147, 1981

Page CP, Carlton PK, Andrassy RJ: Safe, cost-effective post-operative nutrition: Defined formula diet via needle-catheter jejunostomy. Am J Surg 138:939, 1979

Roslyn JJ, Pitt HA, Mann LL, et al: Gallbladder disease in patients on long-term parenteral nutrition. Gastroenterology 84:148, 1983

Viart P: Hemodynamic findings during treatment of protein-calorie malnutrition. Am J Clin Nutr 31:911, 1978

Wagman LD, Burt ME, Brennan MF: The impact of total parenteral nutrition on liver function tests in patients with cancer. Cancer 49:1249, 1982

Wolfe RR, O'Donnell TF, Stone MD, et al: Investigation of factors determining the optimal glucose infusion rate in total parenteral nutrition. Metabolism 29:892, 1980

2

Blood Component Therapy

The ability to separate a unit of whole blood into its various components allows the physician to administer only those components needed by the patient. This approach minimizes side effects from the use of unnecessary components and enables several patients to benefit from a single unit of whole blood (Table 2-1).

BLOOD COMPONENTS

PACKED RED BLOOD CELLS

One unit of packed red blood cells (PRBC) contains 200 ml red blood cell mass (RBCM) in a total volume of 250–350 ml. A 3% increase in the hematocrit of a nonbleeding 70-kg adult is seen after the infusion of a single PRBC unit. The shelf life of PRBC is 21 days and 35 days if citrate phosphate dextrose adenine (CPDA) is used as anticoagulant.

Since PRBC have the same RBCM as whole blood, it provides the same oxygen-carrying capacity, but in a smaller volume. The decrease in volume reduces the possibility of circulatory overload and cardiovascular failure. The removal of plasma also reduces the amount of citrate, sodium, potassium, and ammonia, rendering PRBC superior to whole blood for transfusion to patients with cardiac, renal, or hepatic disease.

The risk of hepatitis after the transfusion of 1 unit of PRBC is the same as for whole blood. PRBC contain all the platelets and white blood cells (WBC) present in the original whole blood unit. Therefore, sensitization to these blood components may occur. If long-term platelet or granulocyte transfusions are anticipated, leukocyte-poor PRBC or frozen-thawed red blood cells (RBC) should be used.

TABLE 2-1. BLOOD COMPONENTS

Component	ml/unit	Shelf Life	Hepatitis Risk
Packed red blood cells (with CPDA-1)	250–350	21 days 35 days	Yes
Leukocyte-poor PRBC	200–250	24 hours	Yes
Frozen PRBC	300	24 hours	Yes
Leukocyte concentrates	300	24 hours	Yes
Platelets (random donor)	30–40	7 days	Yes
Fresh-frozen plasma	250	6 hours	Yes
Cryoprecipitate	15	4 hours	Yes
Albumin 5% 25%	250 50		No

LEUKOCYTE-POOR PRBC

One unit of leukocyte-poor PRBC contains 185 ml of PRBC in a total volume of 200–250 ml. Saline-washed RBC have less than 10% of the original unit's leukocytes, plasma, and platelets. The shelf life of saline-washed RBC is 24 hours. The risk of transfusion-related hepatitis is the same as for whole blood.

Leukocyte-poor PRBC are indicated in patients with previous febrile reactions to PRBC and in patients expected to need long-term platelet or granulocyte transfusion.

FROZEN PRBC

By adding a cryoprotective agent, usually glycerol, RBC can be frozen and stored up to 3 years at $-65°C$. After thawing, the cryoprotective agent and anticoagulant are removed by saline washes. The washing process also removes most leukocytes, platelets, microaggregates, and damaged RBC. One unit of frozen-thawed PRBC contains 170–190 ml of PRBC in 300 ml total volume.

The shelf life after thawing is 24 hours. The risk of transfusion-related hepatitis is the same as for whole blood. Because of its long storage capability, frozen PRBC are indicated for rare blood types and autologous transfusions. Although frozen-thawed PRBC have minimal WBC and platelets, its cost precludes routine use in patients needing leukocyte-poor PRBC.

LEUKOCYTE CONCENTRATES

Leukocyte concentrates are obtained from a single donor by filtration or centrifugation techniques. Units obtained by filtration contain 2–3 × 10^{10} granulocytes, 4 × 10^{10} platelets, and 5–30 ml RBC. Units obtained by centrifugation contain 0.5–2 × 10^{10} granulocytes, 4–7 × 10^{11} platelets, 25–50 ml RBC, and a variable number of lymphocytes. The final product is suspended in 300 ml of citrated anticoagulated plasma solution. The shelf life is 24 hours. The risk of hepatitis is similar to that seen with whole blood.

Granulocyte transfusions are indicated in septic neutropenic patients (less than 500 neutrophils/mm^3) who are unresponsive to adequate antibiotic therapy and whose bone marrow function is not expected to recover within 48 hours. Leukocyte transfusions are rarely used in gynecologic oncology.

Leukocyte concentrates must be ABO-group and Rho(D) compatible. Because of their short circulating half-life (6–12 hours), leukocytes need to be transfused daily. An ordinary blood filter is used. Daily transfusions continue until the infection has subsided or the bone marrow has recovered.

Transfusion-associated urticaria, fever, and chills are frequent. Slight pulmonary insufficiency can also occur. If these occur, the transfusion is continued at a slower rate. Prednisone 20 mg PO and diphenhydramine hydrochloride (Benadryl) 50 mg PO given 30 minutes before the transfusion will lessen the severity of reactions.

PLATELETS

One unit of random donor platelet concentrate contains at least 5.5 × 10^{10} platelets and a few RBC in 30–50 ml of plasma. Platelets have a shelf life of 7 days. The risk of hepatitis is similar to that seen with whole blood. Compatibility testing is not required, but Rh-negative women with reproductive potential should receive Rh-negative units.

In gynecologic oncology, platelet transfusions are used for patients with chemotherapy- or radiotherapy-induced thrombocytopenia and for patients receiving massive blood transfusions.

A 1-hour posttransfusion platelet count should be obtained. One unit of platelets results in a platelet count increment of approximately 7,000/mm^3 in the 70-kg adult who does not have a condition causing rapid platelet destruction. Patients who have received multiple platelet or PRBC transfusions may develop antiplatelet antibodies. Less than the expected increase in the platelet count or a decrease may be seen in these patients. Single-donor HLA-compatible platelets are used in patients sensitized to HLA platelet antigens. One unit of single donor platelets contains 7–10 times the number of platelets in a random donor unit.

FRESH-FROZEN PLASMA (SINGLE DONOR)

A unit of fresh-frozen plasma (FFP) contains 400–500 mg of fibrinogen; 0.7–1.0 activity unit of clotting factors II, V, VII, VIII, IX, X, XI, XII, XIII; and 250 ml of anticoagulated plasma. FFP may be stored up to 1 year at −18°C or colder. The shelf life after thawing is 6 hours. The plasma should be from blood ABO-group compatible with the recipient's RBC.

There is a risk of hepatitis transmission, allergic reaction, fever, chills, and circulatory overload. In gynecologic oncology, FFP is used in patients undergoing massive blood replacement with stored blood (see the section *Indications, bleeding*) It can also be used for rapid reversal of oral anticoagulant therapy. It should not be used as a volume expander because of the risk of hepatitis transmissions.

COAGULATION FACTORS
Cryoprecipitate

Each unit of cryoprecipitate contains 200 mg of fibrinogen, 80 U of factor VIII, 30% factor XIII, and 40–70% von Willebrand factor. It can be stored up to 1 year at −18°C. The shelf life after thawing is 4 hours. Viral hepatitis transmission and allergic and febrile reactions can occur. Compatibility testing is not necessary. Cryoprecipitate is used to treat fibrinogen deficiency and specific clotting factor deficiencies. Approximately 10 U of cryoprecipitate is needed to increase the patient's serum fibrinogen by 100 mg/dl.

Other Factors

Purified factor VIII concentrates and factor IX complex (factors II, VII, IX, and X) are available for the treatment of specific hematologic disorders. While cryoprecipitate is obtained from a single donor, the purified factors are obtained from pooled plasma. Thus, the risk of hepatitis transmission is greater.

ALBUMIN

Normal serum albumin is available as a 250-ml 5% albumin solution in saline (145 mEq/L of sodium) or as a 50-ml, 25% albumin solution in distilled water. It is obtained from chemically processed heat-treated pooled plasma. Albumin transfusions have no hepatitis transmission risk. Circulatory overload, urticaria, fever, and chills can occur. Albumin is used as a volume expander in the presence of hypoproteinemia.

INFUSION GUIDELINES

Only normal saline (0.9% NaCl) should be used with blood components. Hypotonic solutions, e.g., 5% dextrose in water (D_5W), can cause hemolysis. Calcium containing solutions (Ringer's lactate) can initiate in vitro coagulation of citrated blood. Medications are never added to a blood unit. All blood products are administered through a filter that traps particles larger than 160 μm (blood clots, coagulant debris). RBC should be administered through a large-bore catheter or needle (at least 18-gauge). The unit should be manually mixed before administration and every 15 minutes to prevent RBC sedimentation at the outlet port. A new filter and IV tubing are used for each component unit.

An approved blood warmer is used when multiple transfusions

at a rate exceeding 50 ml/min are given or when blood is administered to patients with cold agglutinins active in vitro at 37°C. Approved blood warmers have a visible thermometer and an audible warning signal. The blood is warmed to 37°C. Temperatures above 40°C cause RBC injury. Warming the whole unit of blood by immersion in hot water or with microwave blood warmers is not recommended, since hemolysis will occur with overheating. A unit of blood that is not used after warming must be returned to the blood bank and discarded.

INDICATIONS

CHEMOTHERAPY

Patients receiving chemotherapy for gynecologic malignancies frequently require blood component therapy. The most frequently used components in our specialty are PRBC and platelets.

PRBC

Transfusions of PRBC are administered when the hematocrit is less than 25% or in the symptomatic patient with a hematocrit of 25–30%. Multiple transfusions with PRBC may cause sensitization to platelet and WBC antigens. Leukocyte-poor PRBC should be used if long-term platelet or granulocyte transfusions are anticipated or in patients with previous febrile reactions to PRBC.

PLATELETS

Adequate hemostasis is seen with platelet counts over 100,000/mm^3 and normal platelet function. Platelet transfusions to patients with platelet counts of 20,000–100,000/mm^3 are reserved for those who are actively bleeding. Because of the risk of serious spontaneous hemorrhage, prophylactic platelet transfusions are given when the platelet count falls below 20,000/mm^3. The usual dose for an adult whose platelet count is below 20,000/mm^3 is 6 to 8 units of random donor platelet concentrate. A 1-hour posttransfusion platelet count should be more than 50,000/mm^3. An inadequate increase or a decrease in the platelet count is seen in patients with platelet HLA antibodies. These patients need single-donor HLA-compatible platelets.

In the sensitized patient whose platelet count drops even after the administration of single-donor platelets, further platelet transfusions are reserved for the control of active bleeding. An effort should be made to find a perfect HLA match.

Urticaria, fever, and chills can occur while transfusing platelets. Symptoms may be reduced by slowing the infusion rate and administering 50 g of diphenhydramine hydrochloride (Benadryl) IV, and antipyretics. Future transfusions should be preceded by 20 mg PO of prednisone and 50 mg PO of Benadryl 30 minutes before the transfusion.

Leukocytes

Granulocyte transfusions are rarely used in gynecologic oncology. They have been shown to be effective in reducing mortality from gram-negative sepsis in neutropenic patients. Granulocytes are indicated in septic neutropenic patients (less than 500 neutrophils/m^3) who are unresponsive to adequate antibiotic and supportive therapy in whom bone marrow function is not expected to recover within 48 hours. Daily transfusions through a standard blood filter are given until resolution of the infection or bone marrow recovery.

Severely immunosuppressed or immunodeficient patients should receive leukocyte concentrates that had been irradiated with 1500–3000 cGy to prevent lymphocyte blastogenesis that can initiate a graft-versus-host reaction.

RADIATION THERAPY

An improved tumor control with irradiation has been demonstrated in patients whose hematocrit is above 30%. Weekly complete hemograms are obtained in patients undergoing radiation therapy. A hematocrit above 30% is maintained with PRBC transfusions.

Other blood component therapy is rarely needed in patients receiving primary radiation therapy. Thrombocytopenia and leukopenia are usually managed by a break in the radiation therapy schedule, awaiting bone marrow recovery. Severe bone marrow depression may be seen in the patient receiving radiation therapy and chemotherapy.

BLEEDING

Response to Hemorrhage

Hematocrit is an unreliable measure of acute blood loss. Massive blood loss may produce a minimal acute decrease in hematocrit. The rate of change in hematocrit varies with the rate of transcapillary refill and amount of fluid resuscitation. Thus, a very low hematocrit suggests significant blood loss or preexisting anemia, while a near-normal hematocrit does not rule out significant blood loss. A nonpregnant woman's blood volume is approximately 7% of the ideal body weight (70 ml/kg). A loss of up to 15% of the total blood volume produces minimal hemodynamic changes.

A loss of 15–30% results in tachycardia (greater than 100), tachypnea (greater than 20), and a decrease in pulse pressure (difference between systolic and diastolic pressures). The systolic pressure is minimally changed. Release of catecholamines produces a rise in peripheral resistance, which results in a higher diastolic pressure and the narrower pulse pressure. This amount of blood loss also produces an abnormal capillary blanch test. This test is performed by depressing the patient's fingernail or hypothenar eminence. In the normal patient, the color returns within 2 seconds after release.

A loss of 30–40% of the blood volume results in the classic signs of inadequate perfusion: marked tachycardia and tachypnea, a fall in systolic blood pressure, oliguria, and changes in mentation.

A greater than 40% blood volume loss results in an immediate life-threatening situation. The patient experiences marked tachycardia, significantly depressed systolic blood pressure, a very narrow pulse pressure (or an unobtainable diastolic pressure), negligible urinary output, and marked central nervous system depression.

Blood Loss Replacement

Blood volume loss of up to 15% should be replaced with an isotonic electrolyte solution (Ringer's lactate) in a 3:1 ratio (for every 100 ml of blood loss, 300 ml of crystalloid solution is given). RBC and crystalloids are administered for losses of greater than 15% of the blood volume. When administering blood products, only normal saline is used in the IV line used for blood component administration (see the section *Infusion Guidelines*). The hemodynamic status of the patient is carefully monitored during volume replacement. The management is modified according to the patient's hemodynamic response.

Compared with colloids, crystalloids leave the circulation relatively rapidly. In cases of massive blood loss, whole blood is preferred. If PRBC are used, albumin will be needed for volume expansion. Nonplasma volume expanders could also be used. Only dextrans and hydroxyethyl starch (Hespan) have proved relatively safe and efficient. Hydroxyethyl starch is preferred.

A dilutional coagulopathy can occur with blood replacement of more than 10 U of blood. If abnormal bleeding develops early in resuscitation, coagulation studies, including prothrombin time (PT), partial thromboplastin time (PTT), and fibrinogen, and a platelet count are obtained. A platelet pack (6 to 8 U of random donor platelets) is administered. If the platelet count confirms platelet depletion, a platelet pack is administered after every 10 U of blood transfused. If diffuse microvascular bleeding continues after platelet correction or if the coagulation studies are abnormal, FFP is indicated. Six or more units of FFP is necessary to cause a rise in clotting factors levels.

Hypocalcemia secondary to massive citrated blood transfusion is rarely a problem. The indiscriminate administration of calcium will result in hypercalcemia. The need for calcium supplementation during massive blood transfusions should be determined by measuring ionized calcium and by monitoring the QT interval.

Calcium administration is indicated in patients receiving more than 100 ml of blood per minute and in patients with inadequate cardiac output despite an adequate preload. Two ml of 10% calcium chloride solution is administered through a separate line.

TRANSFUSION REACTIONS

The identification of the donor blood and the recipient must be accurate to avoid fatal hemolytic transfusion reactions. For early detection of reactions, close monitoring of the patient is necessary. The patient's general appearance, temperature, pulse, blood pressure, and respirations are observed and recorded pretransfusion, 15–20 minutes into the transfusion and posttransfusion. Most transfusion reactions are minor and allergic in nature.

MILD REACTIONS

Mild urticaria and pruritus are managed by slowing the transfusion rate and administering 50 mg of IV Benadryl. If the patient has a prior history of mild reactions, these may be prevented by premedication with Benadryl 50 mg PO 30 minutes before the transfusion.

MODERATE TO SEVERE REACTIONS

Such reactions as anxiety, mild dyspnea, headache, tachycardia, fever, chills, flushing, and urticaria indicate a moderate to severe reaction. Mild urticaria and pruritus that does not respond within 30 minutes to antihistamines is also managed as a moderate to severe reaction.

As soon as a moderate to severe reaction is identified, the transfusion is stopped, and the IV line is kept open with normal saline. The remainder of the donor unit with accompanying administration set and a sample of patient's urine and blood sample are delivered to the blood bank for analysis. The patient is treated with IV antihistamines and oral or rectal antipyretics. In severe cases, IV corticosteroids and epinephrine may be necessary.

In the laboratory, the patient's urine sample is evaluated for the presence of hemoglobin; if positive, the centrifuged sediment is examined microscopically for RBC. The patient's blood sample is examinmed for hemolysis and direct Coombs test. If there is evidence of hemolysis, the patient's pretransfusion and post-transfusion blood samples are retyped and the cross-match repeated. The unused blood component unit is cultured and Gram stained.

If organisms are identified on Gram stain, the patient receives appropriate antibiotic therapy, after samples for aerobic and anaerobic blood cultures are obtained.

Febrile reactions are frequently due to platelets and/or leukocyte antibodies, with treatment being symptomatic with antipyretics. Subsequent transfusions should be with leukocyte—poor PRBC and consideration of premedication with antihistamines and corticosteroids.

LIFE-THREATENING REACTIONS

Anxiety, chest or flank pain, headache, dyspnea, fever, chills, restlessness, tachycardia, hypotension, oliguria, hematuria, unexplained bleeding are signs and symptoms of a life-threatening transfusion reaction. The transfusion is immediately stopped. The IV line is kept open with normal saline. The unused donor unit and a postreaction patient's urine and blood specimen are delivered to the blood bank for immediate testing. Blood is also drawn for culture, platelet count, measurement of fibrinogen, and fibrin-split products.

Bacterial Contamination

The presence of hemolysis and organisms on Gram stain is indicative of septic shock. The patient is aggressively managed with volume expansion and appropriate antibiotics. Corticosteroids should not be used.

Hemolysis

The signs of a serious hemolytic transfusion reaction always occur during the transfusion of the first 100 ml of whole blood or PRBC. The airway is maintained and supplemental oxygen administered.

If disseminated intravascular coagulation (DIC) is present, IV heparin, 20,000 IU, is administered. In the presence of hypovolemia, hypotension is treated with volume replacement (crystalloid or albumin). If blood is needed, freshly cross-matched blood is administered. If the blood volume is deemed to be normal and hypotension persists, vasopressors may be required. Hydrocortisone 100 mg IV is administered. To minimize renal tubular damage, 40 mEq of sodium bicarbonate and 1 L of Ringer's lactate are administered rapidly with 100 ml of 20% mannitol. The patient should be normovolemic before diuresis with mannitol is forced.

SUGGESTED READINGS

Blood Transfusion Therapy: A Physician's Handbook. American Association of Blood Banks, Arlington, VA, 1983

Circular of Information of the Use of Human Blood and Blood Components: American Association of Blood Banks, The American Red Cross, and the Council for Community Blood Centers, 1986

Lichtiger B: Blood component therapy for cancer. CA 27:194, 1977

3

Endometrial Cancer

The endometrium is the most common site of invasive cancer of the female genital tract. It is estimated that in the United States in 1989, 34,000 new endometrial cancer cases will be diagnosed and that 3,000 women will succumb to this disease. Endometrial adenocarcinoma is by far the most frequent histologic type. Endometrial adenocarcinoma is an age-specific disease. The mean and median age at diagnosis is 61 years. The largest numbers of patients are between 50 and 64 years of age. Women at increased risk of endometrial cancer are those who have been exposed to unopposed estrogen stimulation of the endometrium. This may be due to chronic anovulation, exogenous estrogen use, or constitutional factors that produce high levels of endogenous estrogen. Factors associated with the development of endometrial adenocarcinoma include obesity, diabetes mellitus, hypertension, nulliparity, exogenous estrogen, anovulatory syndrome, gallbladder disease, early menarche, and late menopause.

Approximately three-fourths of patients with endometrial cancer have stage I disease at diagnosis. Early detection results from the evaluation of abnormal uterine bleeding. Careful staging and appropriate treatment result in a high cure rate. The 5-year survival rate for patients with stage I endometrial adenocarcinoma is 75%. A better survival is observed in patients with well-differentiated tumors and no myometrial invasion. Fractional dilatation and curettage (D&C) and accurate staging must be performed in all patients before the initiation of therapy.

The prognosis and adjuvant therapy of patients with stage I endometrial carcinoma are determined by the grade of the tumor, depth of myometrial invasion, and the presence of nodal metastases. The best adjuvant therapy for patients with poor-prognosis stage I endometrial carcinoma is yet to be determined; suggested

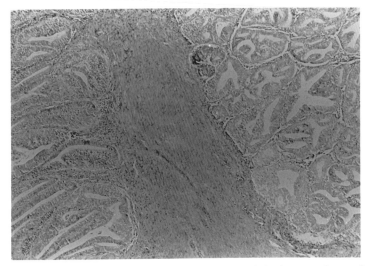

FIG. 3-1. Grade 1 (well-differentiated) endometrial adenocarcinoma invading the myometrium. The glands are back to back with no intervening stroma. There is a gland-in-gland pattern, but there are no solid areas.

guidelines are presented subject to change as new data become available.

HISTOPATHOLOGY

The endometrium is composed of a glandular and a stromal component. Either or both of these components may undergo malignant transformation, giving rise to a variety of tumors. Adenocarcinomas are malignant transformation of the glandular epithelium associated with a benign stroma (Fig. 3-1). They comprise 80–90% of all endometrial cancers. Grading of adenocarcinomas according to the International Federation of Gynecology and Obstetrics (FIGO) is based on architectural patterns (see the section *Staging*). The grade of a tumor is closely associated to the depth of myometrial invasion, lymph node metastasis, and survival. Deep myometrial invasion is present in 10% of grade 1 tumors and in 40% of grade 3 tumors. Lymph node metastasis occurs in 30–40% of patients with deeply invasive tumors and in approximately 3% of those with superficial invasion.

Squamous metaplasia can occur in an endometrial carcinoma. When this metaplasia is benign and associated with a well-differentiated adenocarcinoma, the term adenoacanthoma is used. When the metaplastic squamous epithelium associated with an endometrial adenocarcinoma is malignant, the diagnosis of adenosquamous or adenoepidermoid carcinoma is made. Adenoepidermoid tumors contain an immature squamous element, while adenosquamous tumors contain a mature keratinizing squamous carcinoma. Adenosquamous and adenoepidermoid carcinomas are usually associated with a poorly differentiated glandular component. The prognosis for this type of carcinoma is clearly poorer than for adenocarcinomas.

Other less frequent variants of endometrial adenocarcinoma are the papillary and the clear cell adenocarcinomas. Both variants carry a poorer prognosis. Recently, two types of papillary adenocarcinoma of the endometrium have been identified: the papillary serous adenocarcinoma and the papillary endometrioid adenocarcinoma. The prognosis for patients with papillary endometrioid adenocarcinomas is similar to that for patients with nonpapillary adenocarcinomas, while it is poorer for patients with papillary serous tumors. In a report from Indiana University School of Medicine, Sutton et al. (1987) reviewed 440 patients surgically treated for endometrial adenocarcinoma. Of those with clinical stage I disease, surgical upstaging occurred in 40% of patients with papillary serous tumors compared with 10% in papillary endometrioid and 12.5% in nonpapillary adenocarcinomas.

Pure squamous carcinomas of the endometrium have been reported, but this histologic type is extremely rare. Endometrial stromal sarcomas are uncommon neoplasms of the endometrium in which only the stroma is malignant. Their prognosis is determined by the presence of extrauterine disease, the mitotic activity, and grade of the tumor.

Malignant mixed müllerian (mesodermal) tumors are neoplasms in which both the epithelium and stroma are malignant. The sarcomatous component of heterologous mixed müllerian tumors has tissue not autochthonus to the uterus, e.g., chondrosarcoma, osteosarcoma, liposarcoma, rhabdomyosarcoma. All the tissues in a homologous mixed müllerian tumor, also referred to as carcinosarcomas, are autochthonus to the uterus. Although some investigators have ascribed a poorer prognosis to patients with heterologous mixed müllerian tumors, the prognosis seems to correlate best with the presence or absence of extrauterine tumor.

STAGING

Clinical staging using the FIGO guidelines* is as follows:

Stage 0 Carcinoma in situ. Histologic findings suspicious of malignancy. Cases of stage 0 should not be included in any therapeutic statistics.

Stage I The carcinoma is confined to the corpus (Fig. 3-2).
Stage IA The length of the uterine cavity is 8 cm or less.
Stage IB The length of the uterine cavity is greater than 8 cm.
Stage I cases should be subgrouped according to the histologic degree of differentiation:

  G1 Highly differentiated glandular carcinoma.
  G2 Differentiated glandular carcinoma with partly solid areas.
  G3 Predominantly solid or entirely undifferentiated carcinomas.

Stage II The carcinoma involves the corpus and cervix.

Stage III The carcinoma has extended outside the uterus, but not outside the true pelvis.

Stage IV The carcinoma has extended outside the true pelvis or has obviously involved the mucosa of the bladder or rectum. Bullous edema, as such, does not permit allotment of a case to stage IV.

---

* From Acta Obstet Gynecol Scand 50:1, 1971, with permission.

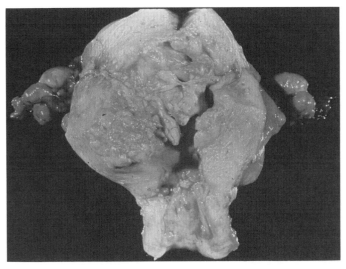

FIG. 3-2. Stage I endometrial adenocarcinoma. Large tumor in the uterine corpus with deep myometrial invasion. Cervix, tubes, and ovaries are grossly free of tumor.

DIAGNOSIS AND PRETREATMENT EVALUATION

DIAGNOSIS

The histopathologic diagnosis of endometrial carcinoma must be confirmed prior to consideration of treatment.

PRETREATMENT EVALUATION

1. Complete medical history and physical examination
2. Complete blood count (CBC)
3. Hepatorenal profile, 2-hour postprandial blood glucose
4. Urinalysis
5. Chest radiograph
6. Excretory urogram (IVP), if computed tomography (CT) scan not done
7. Examination under anesthesia, fractional D&C, and uterine sounding (Fig. 3-3). Since endocervical or frank cervical involvement has a pro-

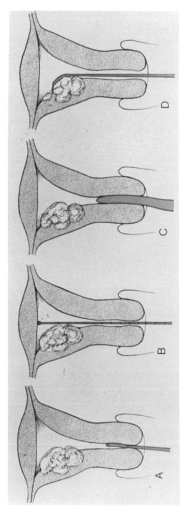

FIG. 3-3. Fractional dilatation and curettage of the uterus. (**A**) Endocervical curettage. (**B**) Uterine sounding. (**C**) Cervical dilatation. (**D**) Endometrial curettage.

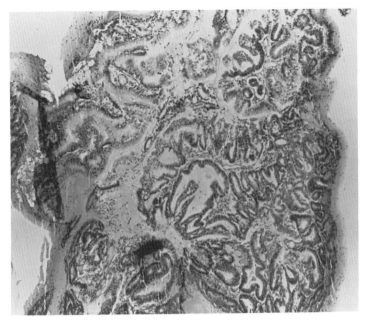

FIG. 3-4. Endocervical curettings from patient with stage II endocervical adenocarcinoma showing normal endocervical glands and endometrial adenocarcinoma.

found effect on staging, treatment, and prognosis, every effort to detect occult cervical involvement should be made. (Fig. 3-4). If fractional curettage has not been previously performed, it should be done before initiating treatment.

8. Cystoscopy and sigmoidoscopy performed for all patients with clinical stage II tumors and beyond
9. Upper gastrointestinal (GI) series and barium enema done as indicated by the patient's symptoms
10. CT scan of the abdomen and pelvis performed for patients with clinical stage II, III, IV and for patients with stage I disease who are to be treated by primary radiation therapy
11. Liver/spleen scan or liver ultrasound if liver enzymes elevated and CT scan not done or equivocal
12. Mammography

GYNECOLOGIC ONCOLOGY TUMOR BOARD

After staging workup, all patients are presented to the Gynecologic Oncology Tumor Board for confirmation of staging. After the patient is clinically staged, a treatment plan is determined.

TREATMENT

STAGE I

The surgical management of patients with stage I disease consists of exploratory laparotomy, peritoneal cytology, total abdominal extrafascial hysterectomy, and bilateral salpingo-oophorectomy. Periaortic and pelvic node sampling is performed in selected

TABLE 3-1. TREATMENT OF STAGE I ENDOMETRIAL ADENOCARCINOMA: EXTRAFASCIAL HYSTERECTOMY, BILATERAL SALPINGO-OOPHORECTOMY, PELVIC AND PERIAORTIC NODE SAMPLING, PERITONEAL WASHINGS

Surgical-Pathologic Findings	Adjuvant Therapy
Grade 1 & 2, with minimal or no invasion	No further treatment
Grade 1 & 2, 50% or less myometrial invasion	7,000 cGy vaginal surface (ovoids or mold)
Grade 1 & 2, more than 50% myometrial invasion	External beam 5,040 cGy total-pelvis to mid-L5 (180 cGy per fraction)
OR	
Adnexal involvement	
OR	
Occult cervical involvement	
OR	
Grade 3	
Positive peritoneal washings	Progestin (Megace)
Positive periaortics	Chemotherapy + Progestin
	OR
	periaortic irradiation (4,500 cGy)

cases with a minimum amount of surgical dissection and manipulation. Any clinically suspicious nodes are removed.

No data have shown an improvement in survival for patients with stage I endometrial adenocarcinoma who underwent pelvic and/or periaortic node dissection. Therefore, the decision to perform node sampling is made after the surgeon experienced in the treatment of this disease weighs the risks and possible benefits. The need for adjuvant radiation therapy is determined on the basis of the histopathologic and cytopathologic findings.

The benefit of adjuvant radiation therapy in different clinical situations is still being defined, an example of which is the patient with a stage I grade 3 tumor with disease confined to the endometrium (e.g., no myometrial invasion). If the peritoneal washings, adnexa, and nodal biopsies are negative, adjuvant therapy may not improve survival. An approach to adjuvant radiation therapy is outlined in Table 3-1.

STAGE II

Patients who are excellent surgical candidates, that is, those patients under 60 years of age who are nonobese and who are neither hypertensive nor diabetic, can be treated by radical abdominal hysterectomy with bilateral pelvic lymph node dissection and periaortic node sampling. If pelvic nodes, aortic nodes, or

TABLE 3-2.   ADJUVANT THERAPY FOR STAGE II
ENDOMETRIAL ADENOCARCINOMA AFTER
RADICAL HYSTERECTOMY

Surgical-Pathologic Findings	Adjuvant Therapy
Positive adnexae	5,000 cGy external beam to mid-L5
Positive pelvic or low common iliac nodes	4,000 cGy external beam to top L4; reduce field to pelvis (mid-L5) for a total of 5,000 cGy
Positive high common iliacs or periaortics with negative scalene fat pad biopsy	4,000 cGy external beam to top L4 and 4,500 cGy to periaortics

adnexae are positive, postoperative irradiation is administered as outlined in Table 3-2.

Most patients with endometrial adenocarcinoma are not candidates for radical surgery and are treated with 4,000 cGy whole-pelvis irradiation (top of L5), a parametrial boost to 4,500 cGy followed by a single radium application using tandem and ovoids for a total of 7,000 cGy to point A (see Fig. 4-3). Four to 6 weeks following this insertion, a total abdominal extrafascial hysterectomy and bilateral salpingo-oophorectomy and periaortic node sampling is performed. If the periaortic nodes are positive, 4,500 cGy is delivered to the periaortic area postoperatively. Patients who are not candidates for any type of surgical therapy are treated definitively with irradiation (see the section *Radiation Treatment of Medically or Technically Inoperable Patients—Stages I, II, and III*).

STAGE III

Patients who have stage III disease by virtue of minimal involvement of the vaginal fornices are treated in the manner described for patients with stage II disease. However, when the vagina is more massively involved or when there is known parametrial involvement, the patient is treated with radiation therapy as described in the section *Radiation Treatment of Medically or Technically Inoperable Patients—Stages I, II, and III.*

STAGE IV

Treatment of patients with stage IV endometrial cancer is individualized. Options include chemotherapy, radiation, and exenteration, if the disease is confined to the pelvis, or a multimodality approach.

PRINCIPLES OF RADIATION THERAPY FOR CARCINOMA OF THE ENDOMETRIUM IN THE POSTOPERATIVE SETTING

VAGINAL IRRADIATION

1. Patients with stage I carcinoma of the endometrium requiring vaginal irradiation are treated 4–6 weeks postoperatively.

2. Vaginal irradiation is done using a vaginal cylinder or ovoids.
3. A dose of 7,000 cGy at the vaginal surface is given in 48–72 hours.
4. Placement of the applicator follows the following guidelines:
    a. Placement is done in the procedure room with appropriate analgesia and sedation.
    b. A thorough pelvic examination is performed.
    c. A Foley catheter is placed and the bulb filled with radiopaque contrast (Renografin).
    d. A surgical clip is placed on the vaginal cuff.
    e. The vaginal cylinder or ovoids are applied.
    f. A radiography is obtained to determine the applicator's position. It should be opposed to the vaginal cuff.
    g. Loading of the radium or cesium is done in the patient's room.
    h. Prophylactic anticoagulation with low-dose heparin or use of sequential pneumatic calf compressor device is advised.
    i. The position of the applicator should be checked at least once every 8 hours.
    j. If the applicator is dislodged and there is a possible missing source, the patient's room should be sealed and radiation safety personnel called.

EXTERNAL IRRADIATION

1. External beam irradiation, if indicated, will commence no sooner than 14 days after the surgical procedure.
2. If whole-pelvis irradiation is to be given, the inferior margin of the field will extend two-thirds the length of the vagina. This distance is determined by inserting a Lucite rod marked in 1-cm intervals into the vagina. A radiograph is taken, and the length of the vaginal tube can be measured. The upper margin of the field will be the midportion of the fifth lumbar vertebra in patients with pelvic or low common iliac nodes and the top of L1 for patients with high common iliac or periaortic nodes.
3. If the field extends beyond the midportion of L5, the dose is calculated at the superior border of the treatment portal; when 4,000 cGy has been delivered to this area, the field is reduced to the mid-L5 level.
4. Patients may be treated with either cobalt-60 or linear accelerator photons. The 10-MeV photons due to their better depth-dose characteristics are the energy of choice.
5. Setting up of the pelvic fields is done using a simulator. The fields are

carefully shaped with lead blocks to minimize the treatment of normal tissue. Weekly portal or image films are obtained to confirm the setup.

RADIATION TREATMENT OF MEDICALLY OR TECHNICALLY INOPERABLE PATIENTS— STAGES I, II, AND III

1. Patients with medically or technically inoperable stage I, II, or III carcinoma of the endometrium are treated by primary radiation therapy alone. A combination of teletherapy (external beam) and brachytherapy (intracavitary radiation) is given when possible.
2. In patients with small uterine cavities, intracavitary radiation is given with tandem and ovoids. When the uterine cavity is large enough to admit at least four Heyman's capsules (uterus will usually be greater than 8 cm in length or will have a central diameter of greater than 1 cm as indicated by probing and rotating the uterine sound), the use of these capsules should be emphasized.
3. The treatment for medically inoperable patients based on stage and grade of tumor is outlined as follows:
   a. *Stage I, grade 1:* 4,000 cGy whole-pelvis external beam radiation and intracavitary radium, for a total of 8,500 cGy to point A (see Fig. 4-3)
   b. *Stage I, grades 2 and 3, and stage II:* 4,000 cGy total pelvis, 600 cGy parametrial boost, and intracavitary radium, for a total of 8,500 cGy to point A
   c. *Stage III:* Treatment tailored to patient's tumor volume distribution
4. The Heyman's capsules used for the treatment of adenocarcinoma of the endometrium are the plastic disposable afterloaded capsules originally described by Simon.
5. The procedure for insertion of Simon afterloading Heyman's capsules is as follows:
   a. Examination under anesthesia
   b. Sterile preparation
   c. Bladder catheterization and inflation of Foley bulb with radiopaque contrast (Renografin)
   d. Placement of gold seeds into cervix
   e. Sounding of endometrial cavity; determination of diameter of cavity by rotation of curved sound

f. Insertion of capsules (fit should be snug, but do not force capsules)
g. Redilatation as necesary if more capsules are required (insert as many capsules as possible)
h. Use of a tandem if four capsules cannot be accommodated
i. Insertion of Fletcher tandem into endocervical canal and Fletcher ovoids in fornices (Simon afterloading ovoids may also be used)
j. Dummy sources inserted and localization films taken first in the operating room to verify placement, then on simulator for computer dosimetry
k. Dose calculations made to rectum, bladder, points A, B, C (common iliacs) and E (external iliacs) (see Fig. 4-3)
l. Loading of sources as described previously for vaginal irradiation (Simon capsules are loaded with cesium sources that are equivalent to radium)

FOLLOW-UP

Patients are examined 4 weeks after surgery or radiation treatment; followed at 3-month intervals for 2 years, and then at 6-month intervals until the fifth anniversary of their treatment. Follow-up will be yearly after 5 years have elapsed. An excretory urogram (IVP) is obtained 1 year after treatment. A CBC, hepatorenal profile, and Papanicolaou smear are obtained at each visit. A chest radiograph is obtained every 6 months.

RECURRENT ENDOMETRIAL CANCER

LOCALIZATION OF SITE OF RECURRENCE

1. Vaginal
2. Pelvis and/or lymph nodes
3. Distant

EVALUATION OF EXTENT OF DISEASE

1. Histopathologic or cytopathologic proof of recurrence and estrogen/progesterone receptors whenever possible
2. CBC, hepatorenal profile

3. Chest radiograph
4. CT scan of abdomen and pelvis
5. Bone scan if alkaline phosphatase is elevated and/or patient has bone pain
6. Upper and lower GI contrast studies if indicated by signs, symptoms, and physical examination
7. Cytoscopy and proctosigmoidoscopy
8. Paracentesis and/or thoracentesis in the presence of fluid

DISPOSITION

After careful evaluation, patients with recurrent endometrial cancer are presented to the Gynecologic Oncology Tumor Board for treatment disposition.

TREATMENT

1. In patients with local or pelvic recurrences in whom no adjuvant vaginal or pelvic radiation therapy was given, whole-pelvis and vaginal radiation can be used. Local excision of vaginal lesions prior to radiation can be attempted. Chemotherapy is used in patients with prior radiation.
2. The patient with documented distant metastases is treated with chemotherapy (see Ch. 7)

SUGGESTED READINGS

Bedwinek J, Galakatos A, Camel M, et al: Stage I, grade III adenocarcinoma of the endometrium treated with surgery and irradiation: Sites of failure and correlation of failure with irradiation technique. Cancer 54:40, 1984

Chambers JT, Merino M, Kohurn EI, et al: Uterine papillary serous carcinoma. Obstet Gynecol 69:109, 1987

Creasman WT, Morrow CP, Bundy BN, et al: Surgical pathologic spread patterns of endometrial cancer. Cancer 60:2035, 1987

Damewood MD, Rosenshein NB, Grumbine FC, et al: Cutaneous metastasis of endometrial carcinoma. Cancer 46:1471, 1980

Davies JL, Rosenshein NB, Antunes CMF, et al: A review of the risk factors for endometrial carcinoma. Obstet Gynecol Surv 36:107, 1981

Demopoulos RI, Dubin N, Noumoff J, et al: Prognostic significance of squamous differentiation in Stage I endometrial adenocarcinoma. Obstet Gynecol 68:245, 1986

Dinh TV, Woodruff JD: Leiomyosarcoma of the uterus. Am J Obstet Gynecol 144:817, 1982

Evans HL, Endometrial stromal sarcoma and poorly differentiated endometrial sarcoma. Cancer 50:2170, 1982

Feuer GA, Calanog A: Endometrial carcinoma: Treatment of positive paraaortic nodes. Gynecol Oncol 27:104, 1987

Genest P, Drouin P, Girard A, et al: Stage III carcinoma of the endometrium: A review of 41 cases. Gynecol Oncol 26:77, 1987

Hernandez E, Rosenshein NB, Dillon MB, et al: Peritoneal cytology in stage I endometrial cancer. J Natl Med Assoc 77:799, 1985

Katz L, Merino MJ, Sakamoto H, et al: Endometrial stromal sarcoma: A clinicopathologic study of 11 cases with determination of estrogen and progestin receptor levels in three tumors. Gynecol Oncol 26:87, 1987

Kennedy AW, Peterson GL, Becker SN, et al: Experience with pelvic washings in stage I and II endometrial carcinoma. Gynecol Oncol 28:50, 1987

Komaki R, Cox JD, Hartz AJ, et al: Prognostic significance of interval from preoperative irradiation to hysterectomy for endometrial carcinoma. Cancer 58:873, 1986

Larson DM, Copeland LJ, Gallagher HS, et al: The significance of residual tumor after preoperative pelvic irradiation for Stage II endometrial carcinoma. Obstet Gynecol 70:916, 1987

Larson DM, Copeland LJ, Gallagher HS, et al: Stage II endometrial carcinoma: Results and complications of combined radiotherapeutic–surgical approach. Cancer 61:1528, 1988

Lifshitz S, Schauberger CW, Platz CA, et al: Primary squamous cell carcinoma of the endometrium. J Reprod Med 26:25, 1981

Lotocki R, Rosenshein NB, Grumbine F, et al: Mixed mullerian tumors of the uterus: Clinical and pathologic correlations. Int J Gynecol Obstet 20:237, 1982

Mackillop WJ, Pringle JF: Stage III endometrial carcinoma: A review of 90 cases. Cancer 56:2519, 1985

Marchetti DL, Piver MS, Tsukada Y, et al: Prevention of vaginal recurrence of Stage I endometrial adenocarcinoma with postoperative vaginal radiation. Obstet Gynecol 67:399, 1986

Mazurka JL, Krepart GV, Lotocki R: Prognostic significance of positive peritoneal cytology in endometrial carcinoma. Am J Obstet Gynecol 158:303, 1988

Piver MS, Rutledge FN, Copeland L, et al: Uterine endolymphatic stromal myosis: A collaborative study. Obstet Gynecol 64:173, 1984

Patanaphan V, Salazar OM, Chougule P: What can be expected when radiation therapy becomes the only curative alternative for endometrial cancer? Cancer 55:1462, 1985

Potish RA, Twiggs LB, Adcock LL, et al: Paraaortic lymph node radiotherapy in cancer of the uterine corpus. Obstet Gynecol 65:251, 1985

Ramirez-Gonzalez CE, Adamsons K, Mangual-Vazquez TY, et al: Papillary adenocarcinoma in the endometrium. Obstet Gynecol 70:212, 1987

Shimm DS, Wang CC, Fuller AF Jr, et al: Management of high-grade stage I adenocarcinoma of the endometrium: Hysterectomy following low-dose external beam pelvic irradiation. Gynecol Oncol 23:183, 1986

Simon N, Silverstone SM: Intracavitary radiotherapy of endometrial cancer by afterloading. Gynecol Oncol 1:13, 1972

Sorbe B: Radiotherapy and/or chemotherapy as adjuvant treatment of uterine sarcomas. Gynecol Oncol 20:281, 1985

Stokes S, Bedwinek J, Breaux S, et al: Treatment of stage I adenocarcinoma of the endometrium by hysterectomy and irradiation: Analysis of complications. Obstet Gynecol 65:86, 1985

Sutton GP, Brill L, Michael H, et al: Malignant papillary lesions of the endometrium. Gynecol Oncol 27:294, 1987

van Nagell JR Jr, Hanson MB, Donaldson ES, et al: Adjuvant vincristine, dactinomycin, and cyclophosphamide therapy in stage I uterine sarcomas. Cancer 57:1451, 1986

Wait RB: Megestrol acetate in the management of advanced endometrial carcinoma. Obstet Gynecol 41:129, 1973

Wallin TE, Malkasian GD Jr, Gaffey TA, et al: Stage II cancer of the endometrium: A pathologic and clinical study. Gynecol Oncol 18:1, 1984

Yamashina M, Kobara TY: Primary squamous cell carcinoma with its spindle cell variant in the endometrium: A case report and review of the literature. Cancer 57:340, 1986

4

Cervical Cancer

The incidence of cervical cancer has decreased markedly over the past three decades. The introduction of the Papanicolaou smear and the identification and treatment of cervical intraepithelial neoplasia are largely responsible for this decreased incidence. It is estimated that in the United States in 1989, 13,000 women will be diagnosed with invasive cervical cancer and more than 50,000 with carcinoma in situ. It is apparent that the most important risk factor is promiscuity. Infection of the cervix with certain types of the human papillomavirus (e.g., 16, 18, 31, 33) is strongly associated with the development of cervical neoplasia.

In 1988 an estimated 7,000 women will die in the United States of cervical cancer. The 5-year survival of patients with cervical carcinoma after treatment is as follows:

Stage	5-Year Survival (%)
I	92
IIA	84
IIB	67
IIIA	45
IIIB	36
IV	14

The pattern of spread of invasive cervical carcinoma is well known. Initial local spread is followed by progressive and orderly nodal metastases. Metastasis to the pelvic lymph nodes is followed by involvement of the periaortic, thoracic, and supraclavicular nodes. A rare case of periaortic node metastasis without pelvic node involvement has been reported. The frequency of lymph node metastases by stage is as follows:

Stage	Nodal Metastasis (%)
I	15–20
II	20–40
III	50

Despite local control, recurrence and death from cervical carcinoma occur from failure of control in the regional and geographic areas of tumor spread. The reported frequency of lymph node metastases to the periaortic nodes by stage is as follows:

Stage	Nodal Metastasis (%)
I	6
IIa	7
IIb	20
III	25
IV	75

Invasive carcinoma of the cervix is both a preventable and a curable disease. Since the pattern of spread is well known, an accurate evaluation of the extent of disease is possible. Factors that should be addressed in the workup and treatment planning of each case include age, previous medical and surgical history, Papanicolaou smear history, anesthetic risk, vaginal distortion, extent of tumor involvement, and potential risks/complications of the planned treatment course. In early stage disease (I and IIA), either primary surgical intervention or therapeutic irradiation is employed. Stages IIB, III, and IV are treated primarily with radiation therapy. Tumoricidal doses of radiation are applied using a combination of external beam therapy and intracavitary irradiation with an accurate dose distribution around the known tumor volume.

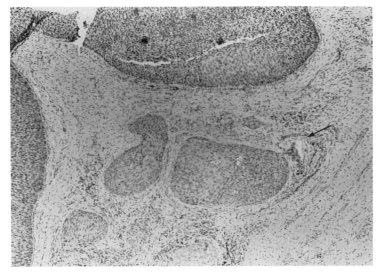

FIG. 4-1. Microinvasive squamous cell carcinoma of the cervix with pre-formed space invasion at arrow. This patient was treated with radical abdominal hysterectomy and bilateral pelvic lymph-adenectomy.

HISTOPATHOLOGY

Squamous cell (epidermoid) carcinoma is the most frequent histologic type of invasive cervical cancer (Fig. 4-1). Investigators at the Mallinckrodt Institute of Radiology reported that 787 (93%) of 849 patients treated for cervical cancer between 1959 and 1977 had epidermoid cancers. Recently, an increase in the proportion of glandular carcinomas of the uterine cervix was noted. The experience at Tripler Army Medical Center was that of 189 women treated for invasive cervical cancer between 1972 and 1985, 35 (19%) had glandular carcinomas (adenocarcinoma/adenosquamous). This increase in the proportion of glandular tumors is believed to be the result of cytologic screening, which detects preinvasive squamous lesions. Treatment of these lesions has lowered the total number of invasive squamous cell carcinomas, while a similar decrease has not been seen among the glandular cancers. At Tripler Army Medical Center, 26% of patients with cervical

TABLE 4-1. FIVE-YEAR SURVIVAL OF WOMEN
WITH CERVICAL ADENOCARCINOMA TREATED AT
THE UNIVERSITY OF CALIFORNIA, LOS ANGELES,
AND AT THE UNIVERSITY OF MARYLAND

Stage	Survival (%)	
	UCLA[a]	UM[b]
I	82	77
II	57	64
III	28	27
IV	0	0

[a] Berek et al. (1981).
[b] Prempree et al. (1985).

cancer who had regular Papanicolaou smears were found to have glandular tumors, as compared with 9% of those not participating in a screening program.

The 5-year survival of women with cervical adenocarcinoma is poorer than that of women with squamous lesions (Table 4-1). The reasons for this are not clear, but several explanations have been advanced: (1) the relative radioresistance of adenocarcinomas; (2) earlier access to lymphatics and capillaries, since glandular tumors begin deeper in the cervix than do squamous tumors; and (3) glandular carcinomas go undetected for longer periods of time.

A number of other histologic types (e.g., adenoid cystic, adenoid basal, clear cell, glassy cell, papillary, small cell, carcinosarcoma) are infrequently found in patients with invasive cervical cancer. A discussion of all these histologic types is beyond the scope of this manual.

STAGING

Clinical staging using the International Federation of Gynecology and Obstetrics (FIGO) guidelines* is as follows:

---

* From Acta Obstet Gynecol Scand 50:1, 1971 and Gynecol Oncol 25:383, 1986, with permission.

PREINVASIVE CARCINOMA

Stage 0 Carcinoma in situ. Cases of stage 0 should not be included in any therapeutic statistics.

INVASIVE CARCINOMA

Stage I The carcinoma is strictly confined to the cervix (extension to the corpus should be disregarded).

Stage IA Preclinical carcinomas of the cervix, that is, those diagnosed only by microscopy.

Stage IA1 Minimal microscopically evident stromal invasion.

Stage IA2 Lesions detected microscopically that can be measured. The upper limit of the measurement should not show a depth of invasion of more than 5 mm taken from the base of the epithelium, either surface or glandular, from which it originates, and a second dimension, the horizontal spread, must not exceed 7 mm. Larger lesions should be staged as IB.

Stage IB Lesions of greater dimensions than stage IA2 whether seen clinically or not. Preformed space involvement should not alter the staging but should be specifically recorded so as to determine whether it should affect treatment decisions in the future.

Stage II The carcinoma extends beyond the cervix but has not extended onto the pelvic wall; it involves the vagina, but not the lower third.

Stage IIA No obvious parametrial involvement.

Stage IIB Obvious parametrial involvement.

Stage III The carcinoma has extended on to the pelvic wall. On rectal examination, there is no cancer free space between the tumor and the pelvic wall. The tumor involves the lower third of the vagina. All cases with hydronephrosis or nonfunctioning kidney that are secondary to the cancer.

Stage IIIA Involvement of the lower third of the vagina. No extension onto the pelvic wall.

Stage IIIB Extension onto the pelvic wall and/or hydronephrosis or nonfunctioning kidney.

Stage IV The carcinoma has extended beyond the true pelvis or has clinically involved the mucosa of the bladder or rectum. Bullous edema as such does not permit a case to be allotted to stage IV.

State IVA   Spread of the growth to the adjacent organs.
Stage IVB   Spread to distant organs.

PRETREATMENT EVALUATION

Objectives in the evaluation of women with invasive cervical carcinoma include the following:

1. Histopathologic documentation of the lesion
2. Evaluation of the patient in preparation for therapy to include medical consultation, pulmonary function testing, arterial blood gases, and other tests and consults as indicated
3. Establishment of the tumor volume and the FIGO stage of the carcinoma
4. Ascertainment of the psychosocial impact of the disease on the patient and her family; consultation with the social worker encouraged
5. Presentation to the Gynecologic Oncology Tumor Board, after the above have been fulfilled, for staging confirmation and recommendations. A note should be written by the house officer in the patient's hospital chart documenting the recommendations of the Tumor Board.

Tests used in determining the FIGO stage include the following:

1. Physical examination with examination under anesthesia if necessary
2. Chest radiograph
3. IVP (excretory urogram)
4. Cystoscopy
5. Proctosigmoidoscopy
6. Bone survey
7. Cytology
8. Histopathology
9. Endocervical curettage
10. Conization if indicated for diagnosis

The above tests should be obtained for every patient, with the exception of the bone survey, which should only be ordered in the symptomatic patient or patient with elevated alkaline phosphatase and normal γ-glutamyl transferase (GGT). These tests fulfill the metastatic workup required on patients with early Stage I cervical carcinoma who are surgical candidates.

The following tests should be obtained on all other patients with invasive cervical cancer:

1. Abdominopelvic CT scan
2. Bone scan if symptomatic or elevated alkaline phosphatase and normal 5′-nucleotidase or GGT
3. Retroperitoneal periaortic node sampling for patients with stage IIB and above (see p. 44)
4. Scalene fat pad biopsy if retroperitoneal exploration demonstrates positive periaortic lymph nodes confirmed by frozen section, (10–30% will show microscopic involvement)

TREATMENT

THERAPY FOR INVASIVE CARCINOMA CONFINED TO THE CERVIX

Definitive therapy for this tumor must encompass the primary carcinoma with an adequate margin of normal tissue. For stages IA2 and above, therapy should include the primary lymphatic drainage (e.g., the pelvic lymph nodes).

There are two primary therapeutic modalities:

1. *Surgery:* Total abdominal extrafascial hysterectomy with or without bilateral pelvic lymphadenectomy for patients with stage IA1, and stage IA2 without lymphovascular invasion; radical abdominal hysterectomy and bilateral pelvic lymphadenectomy for patients with stage IA2 with lymphovascular invasion, stage IB or early IIA; bilateral salpingo-oophorectomy considered in women with glandular carcinomas (e.g., adenocarcinoma, adenosquamous)
2. *Radiotherapy:* External beam via cobalt or linear accelerator and brachytherapy (e.g., radium or cesium implants)

Surgery is generally reserved for patients who are good operative candidates and who have early disease (e.g., not beyond

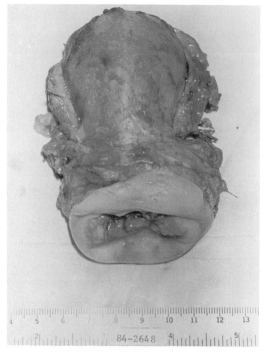

FIG. 4-2. Radical hysterectomy specimen of a patient with stage IIA cervical cancer with minimal involvement of the vaginal fornices with tumor.

early stage IIA) (Fig. 4-2). Since radiation may be used for these patients and is equally effective, the pros and cons of both modalities should be presented to the patient. All other patients are treated with radiation therapy.

Improved survival is seen when patients with stage IB squamous cell carcinoma with a lesion 6 cm or greater in diameter (barrel lesion) are treated with preoperative irradiation (6,000–6,500 cGy to point A) (Fig. 4-3), followed in 4–6 weeks by a total abdominal extrafascial hysterectomy.

The same holds true for patients with stage IIA adenocarcinoma. The best survival for patients with stage IB cervical aden-

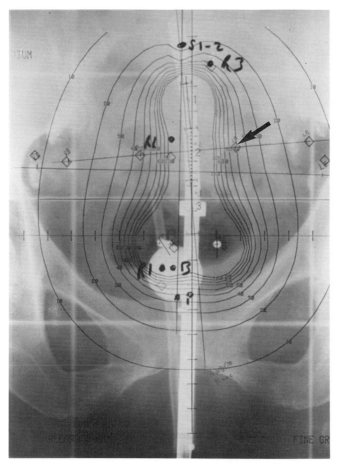

FIG. 4-3. Isodose curve for a radium intracavitary implant using a Fletcher-Suit applicator. R1, R2, and R3 represent rectal points. The bladder is at B. Point A (at arrow) is 2 cm from the midline of the cervical canal and 2 cm superior to the lateral vaginal fornix and represents the dose to the paracervical triangle. Point B is 3 cm lateral to point A and represents the dose received by the obturator nodes. Contrast from a previous lymphangiogram is still seen in the pelvic lymph nodes.

TABLE 4-2.   TREATMENT PLAN FOR PATIENTS WITH
CERVICAL SQUAMOUS CELL CARCINOMA

Stage	Treatment
IB, IIA	Radical hysterectomy or radiation (4,000 cGy whole pelvis and two radium applications—total dose to point A (8,000–8,500 cGy))
IIA	4,000 cGy whole pelvis, 600–1,500 cGy parametria, and two radium applications
IIB	4,000 cGy whole pelvis, 600–1,500 cGy parametria, and two radium applications
III	5,000 cGy whole pelvis, 600–1000 cGy parametria, and one radium application
IV	Individualize

ocarcinoma is seen with radical hysterectomy or with preoperative irradiation followed by an extrafascial hysterectomy. Radiation alone for the treatment of glandular cervical carcinomas should be reserved for patients with small lesions (less than 2 cm). The treatment plan for patients with cervical squamous cell carcinoma is summarized in Table 4-2.

THERAPY FOR CARCINOMA OF THE CERVIX DISSEMINATED TO LYMPH NODES

Patients in this category may be divided as follows:

1. Positive periaortic lymph nodes with negative scalene fat pad: treated with whole-pelvis irradiation, periaortic irradiation, and brachytherapy (intracavitary irradiation)
2. Positive periaortic lymph nodes with positive scalene fat pad: treated with systemic chemotherapy and with pelvic irradiation, if indicated, for pelvic tumor control

FOLLOW-UP

Patients are examined 4 weeks after surgery or radiation treatment. They are followed at 3-month intervals for 2 years and then at 6-month intervals until the fifth anniversary of their treatment.

Follow-up will be yearly after 5 years have elapsed. An IVP is obtained 1 year after treatment. A CBC, hepatorenal profile, and Papanicolaou smear are obtained at each visit. A chest radiograph is obtained every 6 months.

RECURRENT CERVICAL CANCER

LOCALIZATION OF SITE OF RECURRENCE

1. Central (cervix, parametria, vagina)
2. Regional (pelvic sidewalls)
3. Geographic (disease outside the pelvis)

EVALUATION OF EXTENT OF DISEASE

1. Histopathologic or cytologic proof of recurrence
2. CBC
3. Hepatorenal profile
4. Chest radiograph
5. CT scan of abdomen and pelvis
6. Bone scan if alkaline phosphatase is elevated, GGT is normal, and/or patient has bone pain
7. Upper and lower GI contrast studies if indicated by signs, symptoms, and physical examination
8. Examination under anesthesia, cystoscopy, and proctosigmoidoscopy
9. Biopsy of lesions discovered by any of the above studies

DISPOSITION

After the above examination is completed and the extent of the disease has been determined, the case is presented to the Gynecologic Oncology Tumor Board for treatment planning. The patient will benefit from the expertise of several specialists on this multidisciplinary board, who will come up with the therapeutic modality or combination that will best treat the identified tumor volume.

TREATMENT

Pelvic Recurrence

In patients with a pelvic recurrence initially treated with radical surgery only, whole-pelvis and vaginal irradiation can be given. These patients should be considered for retroperitoneal periaortic node biopsy and possible scalene fat pad biopsy if the periaortic nodes are positive.

If the periaortic nodes are positive, and the scalene fat pad biopsy is free of tumor, the radiation field is extended to include the periaortics (top L1). If the scalene fat pad biopsy is positive, the patient is considered for systemic chemotherapy. Pelvic irradiation can be used in these cases to palliate local symptoms.

Central Recurrence

Patients with central recurrences previously treated with irradiation are candidates for pelvic exenteration (en bloc removal of uterus, bladder, and rectosigmoid), if their psychological and general medical status will allow. The initial step when a patient is undergoing laparotomy for possible pelvic exenteration is careful exploration of the pelvis and abdomen, followed by periaortic node sampling. Only patients with resectable disease confined to the pelvis are candidates for this operation. Approximately one-half of patients explored for possible exenteration are found to have disease outside the pelvis or to have unresectable tumor. Hydronephrosis, leg pain, and/or edema prognosticate unresectability. The 5-year survival of patients with recurrent cervical cancer treated with exenteration is 30–40%. The perioperative mortality is approximately 10%.

Distant Metastases

The patient with documented distant metastases is considered for chemotherapy (see Ch. 7). *Cis*-platinum is the most active agent. The response rate is approximately 30%. Unfortunately, the progression-free interval after an initial response is short.

SUGGESTED READINGS

Allen HH, Nisker JA, Anderson RJ: Primary surgical treatment in one hundred ninety-five cases of stage Ib carcinoma of the cervix. Am J Obstet Gynecol 143:581, 1982

Artman LE, Hoskins WJ, Bibro MC, et al: Radical hysterectomy and pelvic lymphadenectomy for stage Ib carcinoma of the cervix: 21 years experience. Gynecol Oncol 28:8, 1987

Belinson JL, Goldberg MI, Averette HE: Paraaortic lymphadenectomy in gynecologic cancer. Gynecol Oncol 7:188, 1979

Berek JS, Castaldo TW, Hacker NF, et al: Adenocarcinoma of the uterine cervix. Cancer 48:2734, 1981

Berman ML, Lagasse LD, Watring WG, et al: The operative evaluation of patients with cervical carcinoma by an extraperitoneal approach. Obstet Gynecol 50:658, 1977

Bleker OP, Ketting BW, van Wayjen-Eecen B, et al: The significance of microscopic involvement of the parametrium and/or pelvic lymph nodes in cervical cancer stages Ib and IIa. Gynecol Oncol 16:56, 1983

Brand E, Berek JS, Hacker NF: Controversies in the management of cervical adenocarcinoma. Obstet Gynecol 71:261, 1988

Buchsbaum HJ: Extrapelvic lymph node metastases in cervical carcinoma. Am J Obstet Gynecol 133:814, 1979

Burke TW, Heller PB, Hoskins WJ, et al: Evaluation of the scalene lymph nodes in primary and recurrent cervical carcinoma. Gynecol Oncol 28:312, 1987

Cardinale JG, Peschel RE, Gutierrez E, et al: Stage IIIA carcinoma of the uterine cervix. Gynecol Oncol 23:199, 1986

Deppe G, Lubicz S, Galloway BT Jr, et al: Aortic node metastases with negative pelvic nodes in cervical cancer. Cancer 53:173, 1984

Dinh TV, Woodruff JD: Adenoid basal carcinoma of the cervix. Obstet Gynecol 65:705, 1985

Gallion HH, van Nagell JR Jr, Donaldson ES, et al: Combined radiation therapy and extrafascial hysterectomy in the treatment of stage Ib barrel-shaped cervical cancer. Cancer 56:262, 1985

Hernandez E, Miyazawa K, Berenberg J: Cervical adenocarcinoma among cytologically screened and unscreened women. Gynecol Oncol 29:140, 1988 (abst)

Kaminski PF, Maier RC: Clear cell adenocarcinoma of the cervix unrelated to diethylstilbestrol exposure. Obstet Gynecol 62:720, 1983

Kaminski PF, Norris HT: Coexistence of ovarian neoplasms and endocervical adenocarcinoma. Obstet Gynecol 64:553, 1984

Larson DM, Stringer A, Copeland LJ, et al: Stage Ib cervical carcinoma treated with radical hysterectomy and pelvic lymphadenectomy: Role of adjuvant radiotherapy. Obstet Gynecol 69:378, 1987

Mann WJ, Chumas J, Amalfitano T, et al: Ovarian metastases from stage Ib adenocarcinoma of the cervix. Cancer 60:1123, 1987

Montana GS, Fowler WC, Varia MA, et al: Analysis of results of radiation therapy for stage II carcinoma of the cervix. Cancer 55:956, 1985

Montana GS, Fowler WC, Varia MA, et al: Carcinoma of the cervix, stage III: Results of radiation therapy. Cancer 57:148, 1986

Pak HY, Yokota SB, Paladugn RR, et al: Glassy cell carcinoma of the cervix: Cytologic and clinicopathologic analysis. Cancer 52:307, 1983

Perez CA, Breaux S, Madol-Jones H, et al: Radiation therapy alone in the treatment of carcinoma of the uterine cervix. I. Analysis of tumor recurrence Cancer 51:1393, 1983

Potish R, Adcock L, Jones T Jr, et al: The morbidity and utility of periaortic radiotherapy in cervical carcinoma. Gynecol Oncol 15:1, 1983

Prempree T, Amornmarn R, Wizenberg MJ: A therapeutic approach to primary adenocarcinoma of the cervix. Cancer 56:1264, 1985

Randall MC, Kim JA, Mills JE, et al: Uncommon variants of cervical carcinoma treated with radical irradiation: A clinicopathologic study of 66 cases. Cancer 57:816, 1986

Smotkin D, Berek JS, Fu YS, et al: Human papillomavirus deoxyribonucleic acid in adenocarcinoma and adenosquamous carcinoma of the uterine cervix. Obstet Gynecol 68:241, 1986

5

Ovarian Cancer

Ovarian cancer is the second most common gynecologic malignancy and is responsible for more deaths than endometrial and cervical cancer combined. It is estimated in 1989 that 20,000 new cases will have been diagnosed in the United States and that 12,000 women will have died of this disease. The 5-year survival rate for ovarian cancer is 30–40% and has remained relatively constant over the past three decades.

No signs or symptoms are specific for ovarian cancer. The patient may complain of vague gastrointestinal (GI) symptoms, abdominal distention, or discomfort, or she may be asymptomatic and have a pelvic mass detected on a routine gynecologic examination. Ovarian cancer is not infrequently found at the time of exploratory laparotomy done for other indications.

The pattern of presentation may be responsible for 70% of patients having disseminated disease at the time of diagnosis. Similarly, the poor prognosis for these patients could be partially explained by the late stage of the disease at the time of diagnosis.

Epithelial tumors of the ovary account for more than 80% of ovarian malignancies (see the section *Histology*). Epithelial ovarian cancer is an age-specific disease; the typical patient is in the sixth decade of life. Age-specific incidence increases exponentially after age 40 until age 70, when the rate decreases. Age-specific mortality rates exhibit the same kind of trend, except that mortality peaks at age 70–74. It has been postulated that the rise in circulating gonadotrophins at the time of menopause may be associated with the increased incidence in ovarian cancer observed in that age group. Similarly, the rarity of epithelial cancer among children may be attributable to their lack of prolonged exposure to gonadrotropins.

Nulliparity or low parity is strongly associated with epithelial ovarian cancer. Two hypotheses have been advanced to explain this relationship: (1) pregnancy has a protective effect and (2) inherent ovarian dysfunction is responsible for both low fertility and an increased risk of developing ovarian cancer.

Environmental factors also appear to place the patient at increased risk. This is demonstrated by differences in international incidence data and migration studies. For example, the incidence of ovarian cancer is higher among women in industrialized nations, except for Japan. Age-adjusted incidence rates are highest in Sweden and Denmark (15.1/100,000) and lowest in Japan (2.8/100,000.) Rates among Japanese who migrate to United States (Issei and Nisei) approach those of Caucasian Americans (14/100,000). In Israel, rates are higher among immigrants from Europe and America and lower among immigrants from Asia and Africa. Jewish women born in Israel have rates of ovarian cancer that lie somewhere between those exhibited by the two migrant groups. Investigators studying the epidemiology of ovarian cancer have tried to associate it with multiple environmental factors, previous viral infections, hormonal ingestion, and menstrual history. The associations are weak and conflicting. Different from other gynecologic malignancies, laparotomy is necessary to establish the histologic diagnosis and determine the extent of the disease. The staging of ovarian cancer is established by the surgical, histologic, and cytologic findings. Meticulous staging and tumor-reductive surgery are the cornerstone of ovarian cancer therapy.

HISTOPATHOLOGY

The ovary is the site for a variety of neoplasms; thus, ovarian cancer is not one disease, but many. In an attempt to standardize the nomenclature used in describing the various ovarian tumors, the World Health Organization (WHO) devised a classification based on the histogenesis of the different neoplasms. The WHO classification lists nine major groups for benign and malignant tumors (Table 5-1).

Epithelial ovarian neoplasms arise from the mesothelial cells on the ovarian surface and recapitulate the histology of the female genital tract. This group of tumors is responsible for more than

TABLE 5-1. WORLD HEALTH ORGANIZATION
CLASSIFICATION OF OVARIAN TUMORS (MAJOR GROUPS)

   I. Common epithelial tumors
      A. Serous tumors
      B. Mucinous tumors
      C. Endometrioid tumors
      D. Clear cell (mesonephroid) tumors
      E. Brenner tumors
      F. Mixed epithelial tumors
      G. Undifferentiated carcinoma
      H. Unclassified epithelial tumors
  II. Sex cord (gonadal stromal) tumors
      A. Granulosa-stromal cell tumors
      B. Androblastomas; Sertoli-Leydig cell tumors
      C. Gynandroblastoma
      D. Unclassified
 III. Lipid (lipoid) cell tumors
 IV. Germ cell tumors
      A. Dysgerminoma
      B. Endodermal sinus tumor
      C. Embryonal carcinoma
      D. Polyembryoma
      E. Choriocarcinoma
      F. Teratomas
      G. Mixed forms
  V. Gonadoblastoma
      A. Pure
      B. Mixed with dysgerminoma or other form of germ cell tumor
 VI. Soft tissue tumors not specific to ovary
VII. Unclassified tumors
VIII. Secondary (metastatic) tumors
 IX. Tumor-like conditions

(From Serov et al., 1973, with permission.)

80% of all ovarian cancers. The most common histologic type of ovarian cancer is the papillary serous cystadenocarcinoma (Figs. 5-1 and 5-2), which accounts for approximately one-half of all malignant epithelial ovarian tumors. Mucinous cystadenocarcinoma (Figs. 5-3 and 5-4) comprise 13%, clear cell and endometrioid combined 10%, and other unspecified types 27%.

The degree of cellular differentiation of the epithelial ovarian neoplasm expressed as histologic grade has important prognostic

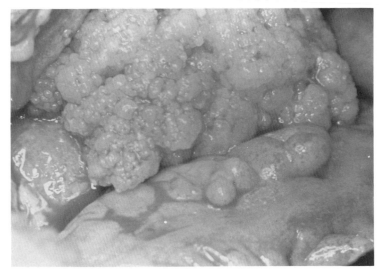

FIG. 5-1. Papillary serous cystadenocarcinoma replacing the right ovary. Note the cauliflower-like appearance of the tumor. The sigmoid colon is at the bottom of the picture, and the uterus is in the left bottom corner.

significance. The criteria used include mitotic count, stratification, cellular pleomorphism, nuclear atypism, and proportion of solid areas within the tumor. Grade 0 tumors (Figs. 5-5 and 5-6), also known as borderline malignancies or tumors of low malignant potential, demonstrate papillary tufting, stratification, epithelial atypia, exfoliation of cellular clusters, minimal mitotic activity, and *no stromal invasion*. The 5-year survival rate of patients with stage I grade 0 tumors is greater than 90%, compared with only a 54% survival for patients with stage I grade 3 serous cystadenocarcinomas. When both stage and grade of epithelial ovarian cancers are the same, there seems to be no significant difference in survival, between histologic cell types.

Significant variability in the interpretation of tumor grade has been found among pathologists. Flow cytometry analysis of tumor DNA content provides another method of assessing tumor differentiation and prognosis. The survival of patients with aneuploid tumors is poorer than that of patients with diploid tumors. The relative risk of death increases with increasing S-phase fraction

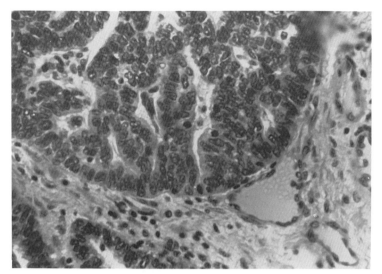

FIG. 5-2. Moderately differentiated ovarian serous cystadenocarcinoma showing numerous mitoses. This tumor recapitulates the histology of the fallopian tube. Differentiation of some cells towards ciliated and secretory cell types can be appreciated.

and higher DNA index. Tumor DNA analysis by flow cytometry is an area of active research with a rapidly expanding fund of information.

Malignant neoplasms of germ cell or stromal origin comprise about 4% of ovarian cancers. The most common histogenetic group of ovarian cancer in patients under the age of 20 are germ cell tumors (dysgerminomas, malignant teratomas, and embryonal carcinomas). These tumors contribute significantly to mortality statistics for children and adolescents.

STAGING

The surgical-pathologic staging according to the International Federation of Gynecology and Obstetrics (FIGO) guidelines* is as follows:

---

* From Gynecol Oncol 25:383, 1986, with permission.

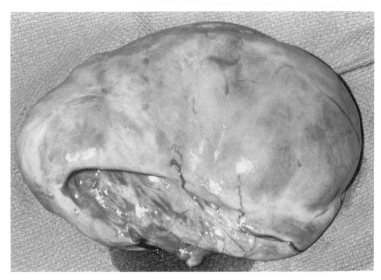

FIG. 5-3. Large mucinous cystadenocarcinoma. In contrast to the serous cystadenocarcinoma (Fig. 5-1), the external capsule of the
mucinous cystadenocarcinoma is usually smooth.

Stage I	Growth limited to the ovaries.
Stage IA	Growth limited to one ovary; no ascites. No tumor on the external surface; capsule intact.
Stage IB	Growth limited to both ovaries; no ascites. No tumor on the external surfaces; capsule intact.
Stage IC	Tumor either stage IA or IB but with tumor on surface of one or both ovaries; or with capsule ruptured; or with ascites present containing malignant cells or with positive perito- neal washings.
Stage II	Growth involving one or both ovaries with pelvic extension.
Stage IIA	Extension and/or metastases to the uterus and/or tubes.
Stage IIB	Extension to other pelvic tissues.
Stage IIC	Tumor either stage IIA or IIB, but with tumor on surface of one or both ovaries; or with capsule(s) ruptured; or with ascites present containing malignant cells or with positive peritoneal washings.

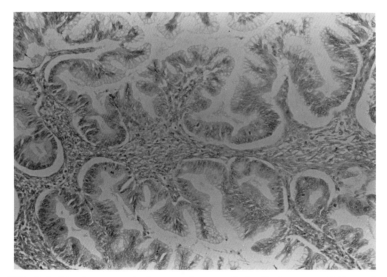

FIG. 5-4. Mucinous cystadenocarcinoma. Note that some of the cells recapitulate the normal histology of the endocervix with the nucleus situated at the base of the cell and the vacuolated cytoplasm towards the lumen. The malignant nature of the above tumor is characterized by finding areas of loss of cellular differentiation (lower left), numerous mitoses, stratification, and a complex glandular pattern.

Stage III	Tumor involving one or both ovaries with peritoneal implants outside the pelvis and/or positive retroperitoneal or inguinal nodes. Superficial liver metastasis equals stage III. Tumor is limited to the true pelvis but with histologically proven malignant extension to small bowel or omentum.
Stage IIIA	Tumor grossly limited to the true pelvis with negative nodes but with histologically confirmed microscopic seeding of abdominal peritoneal surfaces.
Stage IIIB	Tumor of one or both ovaries with histologically confirmed implants of abdominal peritoneal surfaces none exceeding 2 cm in diameter; nodes are negative.
Stage IIIC	Abdominal implants greater than 2 cm in diameter and/or positive retroperitoneal or inguinal nodes.

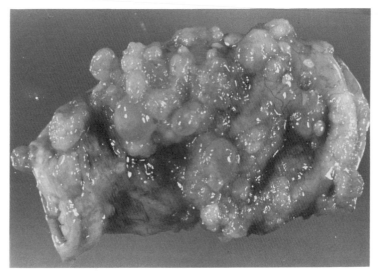

FIG. 5-5. Serous tumor of low malignant potential removed from the right ovary of a 30-year-old woman. The external surface of the tumor was smooth. The tumor was fluid filled, and the inside of the capsule was studded with papillary excrescences.

Stage IV   Growth involving one or both ovaries with distant metastases. If pleural effusion is present, there must be positive cytology to allot a case to stage IV. Parenchymal liver metastasis equals stage IV.

STAGING WORKUP

PRELAPAROTOMY EVALUATION

1. History and physical examination
2. Complete blood count (CBC) with differential, hepatorenal profile
3. Urinalysis
4. Chest radiographs, posterolateral (PA) and lateral
5. Electrocardiogram (ECG)
6. Excretory urogram
7. Thoracentesis mandatory for any patient with a pleural effusion

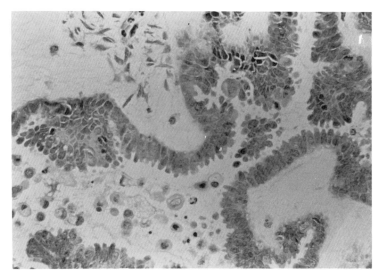

FIG. 5-6. Serous tumor of low malignant potential. There is cellular atypia, stratification, papillary tufting, and 0-1 mitotic figures per high-power field. Atypical cells, single and in clusters, are shed into the lumen.

8. Serum biomarkers: Carcinoembryonic antigen (CEA) α-fetoprotein, human chorionic gonadotropin (hCG), CA-125.
9. Medical consultations as indicated
10. Stool Hemoccult (occult blood test)
11. Radiologic evaluation by computed tomography (CT), upper GI series with small bowel followthrough, barium enema (when clinically indicated)
12. Other diagnostic testing as indicated

STAGING LAPAROTOMY

1. Vertical midline incision: symphysis to midway between umbilicus and xiphoid
2. Peritoneal washings or ascitic fluid for cytology
3. Diaphragm visualized and palpated; washings for cytology using a Robinson catheter to direct the saline to the diaphragm and/or diaphragmatic scrapings taken; biopsies taken of suspicious areas

4. Liver palpated; biopsy obtained of any lesion detected
5. Omentum inspected and an infracolic omentectomy performed
6. All parietal peritoneal surfaces inspected and palpated; biopsies taken of any adhesions and irregularities
7. Random biopsies obtained from the right and left gutters, if no abnormalities observed.
8. Small bowel and its mesentery closely inspected from the ligament of Treitz to the ileocecal valve; biopsies taken from all areas of thickening, adhesions, or irregularities; appendectomy performed
9. Periaortic and pelvic nodes explored and sampled
10. Pelvis carefully explored to determine extent of involvement:
    a. Ovarian capsule intact, smooth, excresences, adhesions
    b. Cystic mass removed atraumatically to avoid rupture and spillage of tumor cells
    c. Biopsies taken of all adherences to pelvic sidewall and surrounding organs
    d. Total abdominal hysterectomy and bilateral salpingo-oophorectomy
    e. Conservative surgery (unilateral salpingo-oophorectomy) considered in the case of a young woman, desirous of childbearing, who has a stage IA well-differentiated cystadenocarcinoma (grade 1) or a tumor of low malignant potential (grade 0); conservative surgery also indicated in a young woman or child with a malignant stage IA germ cell tumor (these tumors are never bilateral, except for dysgerminomas, which are bilateral in 16% of cases); young women with gonadostromal tumors also candidates for conservative surgery
    f. Complete surgical staging required, even if unilateral disease identified; includes biopsy of the contralateral ovary in cases of cystadenocarcinoma or dysgerminoma
    g. Debulking of other tumor masses indicated when it will reduce the tumor volume to a size that will enhance adjuvant therapy, hence survival (residual implants of 2 cm or less)
11. Suspicious inguinal nodes biopsied

DISPOSITION

Following the staging workup and staging laparotomy, the patient is presented to the Gynecologic Oncology Tumor Board for discussion and consideration of adjuvant therapy.

ADJUVANT THERAPY FOR PATIENTS WITH EPITHELIAL OVARIAN CANCER

STAGES

Stage I, grade 1: No further therapy

Stage I, grade 2 and 3: Alternatives include the following:
1. Alkeran, 0.7 mg/m^2 PO everyday for 5 days; repeated every 28 days for at least 6 months.
2. Intraperitoneal chronic phosphate (^{32}P)
3. Cytoxan 1,000 mg/m^2 and *cis*-platinum 100 mg/m^2 every 21 days for three cycles (Gynecologic Oncology Group protocol)

Stages II–IV: Alternatives include the following:
1. Multiagent chemotherapy (e.g., Cytoxan–Adriamycin–Platinol) or inclusion in a research protocol
2. Whole abdominal irradiation is another alternative used in patients with stage II–IIIA disease

SECOND-LOOK LAPAROTOMY

1. This approach is considered only for those patients who have completed the planned chemotherapy courses without clinical evidence of residual or progressive disease and who are being evaluated for termination of therapy.
2. The second surgical exploration is essentially the same as the staging laparotomy. Peritoneal washings are obtained from the pelvis, paracolic gutters, and diaphragm. If no gross tumor is identified, biopsies are obtained of any areas of thickening, adhesions, or irregularities. Random biopsies are obtained for the paracolic gutters, the bladder, and the cul-de-sac peritoneum. The residual omentum is removed. Thorough nodal evaluation is performed. The infundibulopelvic ligaments are biopsied. Biopsies are obtained of areas known to have had residual disease at the time of initial exploration.

RECURRENT PROGRESSIVE DISEASE

1. Patients with persistent or recurrent disease following primary therapy are managed according to
   a. Tumor status (e.g., bulky, diffuse, microscopic)
   b. Location of disease (e.g., pelvis, abdomen, chest).

   c. Manifestation of disease (e.g., pleural effusion, ascites, intestinal obstruction, asymptomatic)

2. Treatment alternatives
    a. Radiation therapy—intraperitoneal radioactive phosphorus (^{32}P) in patients with minimal disease
    b. Alternate chemotherapy protocols (e.g., intraperitoneal cis-platinum)
    c. Hormonal therapy (e.g., Tamoxifen, progestins)
    d. Symptom control
        (1) Thoracentesis and sclerosing agent for pleural effusion
        (2) Repeated paracentesis or Levine shunt for recurrent ascites
        (3) Nasogastric tube or gastrostomy tube to control vomiting
        (4) Pain control

FOLLOW-UP

During therapy, patients are seen at least once a month. A monthly hemogram (CBC), chemistry/liver panel, CA-125, and chest radiograph are obtained. A pelvic examination to assess disease status is done on a monthly basis. Patients receiving chemotherapy have blood drawn for a CBC on days 10–14 of the chemotherapy cycle. Patients receiving whole abdominal irradiation have weekly hemograms.

Patients who have completed therapy and who are free of disease are evaluated every 2–3 months for 2 years. Thereafter, they are evaluated every 6 months. Their evaluation is similar to that undertaken for patients receiving therapy.

THERAPY FOR GERM CELL TUMORS
DYSGERMINOMA

Seventy percent of patients with dysgerminoma have stage I disease at diagnosis with a 5-year survival of 90%. Unilateral salpingo-oophorectomy with adequate surgical staging is the recommended therapy. No adjuvant therapy is necessary. Recurrences are treated with radiation therapy (since dysgerminomas are exquisitely radiosensitive) or by chemotherapy.

Advanced disease (stage II and above) requires total abdominal hysterectomy, bilateral salpingo-oophorectomy, and tumor-reductive surgery. Therapy consists of irradiation or multiagent chemotherapy. The chemotherapy regimens include vincristine—actinomycin D–Cytoxan (VAC) and the modified Einhorn regimen (bleomycin–vinblastine–*cis*-platinum). Regimens that substitute VP-16 (etoposide) for vinblastine, that is, bleomycin–etoposide–*cis*-platinum (BEP), have been found as effective and less toxic (see Ch. 7).

IMMATURE TERATOMA

Most patients with immature teratomas have stage I disease at diagnosis. The prognosis and need for adjuvant therapy is dictated by the stage and grade of the tumor.

Tumor grade is based on the degree of immaturity, presence, and the quantity of neuroepithelium. Survival is related to the grade of the tumor. As demonstrated by Norris and co-workers, the 5-year actuarial survival for patients with grade 1, 2, and 3 neoplasms is 81%, 60%, and 30%, respectively. The actuarial survival for stage I disease, grades 1, 2, and 3, is 100%, 70%, and 33%, respectively.

Patients with stage I disease can be treated with conservative surgery. Chemotherapy (e.g., VAC, modified Einhorn) is recommended for patients with advanced disease (stage II and beyond) and for patients with stage I grade 2 or 3 neoplasms.

ENDODERMAL SINUS TUMOR

Seventy percent of patients with endodermal sinus tumor have stage I disease at diagnosis. No difference in survival is noted when patients with stage I disease are treated with unilateral salpingo-oophorectomy as compared with bilateral salpingo-oophorectomy. The median age of these patients is 19 years. Therefore, conservative surgery is indicated for stage I disease. The survival of patients with endodermal sinus tumor has improved with the addition of adjuvant chemotherapy (e.g., VAC) from 16 to 86%. The modified Einhorn regimen (PVB) or bleomycin–etoposide–*cis*-platinum (BEP) is advocated by some for patients with advanced disease.

FOLLOW-UP FOR PATIENTS WITH GERM CELL TUMORS

Follow-up management for patients with germ cell tumors is similar to that described for patients with ovarian cancer in general. In addition, endodermal sinus tumor produces α-fetoprotein; choriocarcinomas and embryonal carcinomas produce hCG. Some patients with dysgerminomas have markedly elevated lactic dehydrogenase (LDH) (above, 1,000 U/L). These biologic markers are obtained at each visit.

An abdominopelvic CT scan is obtained at the completion of therapy if no second-look laparotomy is contemplated. Thereafter, abdominopelvic CT is obtained every 6 months for 2 years.

SUGGESTED READINGS

Adcock LL: Germ cell tumors of the ovary—Lymph node metastases. Gynecol Oncol 23:234, 1986

Barber HRK: Ovarian cancer: Diagnosis and management. Am J Obstet Gynecol 150:910, 1984

Beecham J, Blessing J, Creasman W, et al: Tamoxifen responsiveness, hormone receptors, and tumor grade: A prospective study of 105 advanced ovarian cancer patients. Gynecol Oncol 29:136, 1988 (abst)

Berek JS, Knapp RC, Malkasian G, et al: CA 125 serum levels correlated with second-look operations among ovarian cancer patients. Obstet Gynecol 67:685, 1986

Burghardt E, Pickel H, Lahousen M, et al: Pelvic lymphadenectomy in operative treatment of ovarian cancer. Am J Obstet Gynecol 155:315, 1986

Chaitin BA, Gershenson DM, Evans HL: Mucinous tumors of ovary: A clinicopathologic study of 70 cases. Cancer 55:1958, 1985

Conte PF, Bruzzone M, Chiara S, et al: A randomized trial comparing cisplatin plus cyclophosphamide versus cisplatin, doxorubicin, and cyclophosphamide in advanced ovarian cancer. J Clin Oncol 4:965, 1986

Coussens PD, Hernandez E, Miyazawa K: Pregnancy after intensive chemotherapy for an ovarian immature teratoma. Milit Med 150:559, 1985

Creasman WT, Park R, Norris H, et al: Stage I borderline ovarian tumors. Obstet Gynecol 59:93, 1982

Dauphlat J, Ferriere J-P, Gorbinet M, et al: Second-look laparotomy in managing epithelial ovarian carcinoma. Cancer 57:1627, 1986

Decker DG, Fleming TR, Malkasian, GD Jr, et al: Cyclophosphamide plus cis-platinum in combination: Treatment program for stage III or IV ovarian carcinoma. Obstet Gynecol 60:481, 1982

Dembo AJ, Bush RS, Beale FA, et al: Ovarian carcinoma: Improved survival following abdominopelvic irradiation in patients with a completed pelvic operation. Am J Obstet Gynecol 134:793, 1979

Einhorn N, Nilsson B, Sjovall K: Factors influencing survival in carcinoma of the ovary: Study from a well-defined Swedish population. Cancer 55:2019, 1985

Fujii S, Konishi T, Suzuki A, et al: Analysis of serum lactic dehydrogenase levels and its isoenzymes in ovarian dysgerminoma. Gynecol Oncol 22:65, 1985

Gallup DG, Talledo OE, Dudzinski MR, et al: Another look at the second-assessment procedure for ovarian epithelial carcinoma. Am J Obstet Gynecol 157:590, 1987

Geisler HE: Megestrol acetate for the palliation of advanced ovarian carcinoma. Obstet Gynecol 61:95, 1983

Gershenson DM, Copeland LJ, Del Junco G, et al: Second-look laparotomy in the management of malignant germ cell tumors of the ovary. Obstet Gynecol 67:789, 1986

Gershenson DM, Copeland LJ, Kavanagh JJ, et al: Treatment of malignant non-dysgerminomatous germ cell tumors of the ovary with vincristine, dactinomycin, and cyclophosphamide. Cancer 56:2756, 1985

Gershenson DM, Del Junco G, Herson J, et al: Endodermal sinus tumor of the ovary: The M.D. Anderson experience. Obstet Gynecol 61:194, 1983

Gershenson DM, Del Junco G, Silva EG, et al: Immature teratoma of the ovary. Obstet Gynecol 68:624, 1986

Gershenson DM, Kavanaugh JJ, Copeland LJ, et al: Treatment of malignant non-dysgerminomatous germ cell tumors of the ovary with vinblastine, bleomycin, and cisplatin. Cancer 57:1731, 1986

Gershenson DM, Wharton JT, Kline RC, et al: Chemotherapeutic remission in patients with metastatic ovarian dysgerminoma: Potential for cure and preservation of reproductive capacity. Obstet Gynecol 58:2594, 1986

Gruppo Interegionale Cooperativo Oncologico Ginecologia: Randomised comparison of cisplatin with cyclophosphamide/cisplatin and with cyclophosphamide/doxorubicin/cisplatin in advanced ovarian cancer. Lancet 2:353, 1987

Hacker NF, Berek JS, Pretorius G, et al: Intraperitoneal cis-platinum as salvage therapy for refractory epithelial ovarian cancer. Obstet Gynecol 70:759, 1987

Heintz APM, Hacker NF, Berek JS, et al: Cytoreductive surgery in ovarian carcinoma: Feasibility and morbidity. Obstet Gynecol 67:783, 1986

Heintz APM, Hacker NF, Lagasse LD: Epidemiology and etiology of ovarian cancer. A review. Obstet Gynecol 66:127, 1985

Hernandez E, Rosenshein NB, Bhagavan BS, et al: Interobserver variability in the interpretation of epithelial ovarian cancer. Gynecol Oncol 17:117, 1984

Hernandez E, Rosenshein NB, Parmley TH: Mucinous cystadenocarcinoma in a premenarchal girl. South Med J 75:1265, 1982

Hernandez E, Rosenshein NB, Villar J, et al: Alternating multiagent chemotherapy for advanced ovarian cancer. J Surg Oncol 2:87, 1983

Ho AG, Bellar U, Speyer JL, et al: A reassessment of the role of second-look laparotomy in advanced ovarian cancer. J Clin Oncol 5:1316, 1987

Hreshchyshyn MM, Park RC, Blessing JA, et al: The role of adjuvant therapy in stage I ovarian cancer. Am J Obstet Gynecol 138:139, 1980

Kallioniemi O-P, Punnonen R, Mattila J, et al: Prognostic significance of DNA index, multiploidy, and S-phase fraction in ovarian cancer. Cancer 61:334, 1988

Krebs H-B, Goplerud DR: Surgical management of bowel obstruction in advanced ovarian cancer. Obstet Gynecol 61:327, 1983

Krebs H-B, Goplerud DR: The role of intestinal intubation in obstruction of the small intestine due to carcinoma of the ovary. Surg Gynecol Obstet 158:467, 1984

Krebs H-B, Goplerud DR, Kilpatrick J, et al: Role of CA 125 as tumor marker in ovarian carcinoma. Obstet Gynecol 67:473, 1986

Kurman RJ, Norris HJ: Malignant germ cell tumors of the ovary. Hum Pathol 8:551, 1977

Lavin PT, Knapp RC, Malkasian G, et al: CA 125 for the monitoring of ovarian carcinoma during primary therapy. Obstet Gynecol 69:223, 1987

Leers WH, Kock HCLV: The evaluation of postoperative irradiation in patients with early-stage ovarian cancer. Gynecol Oncol 28:41, 1987

Malfetano JH: The appendix and its metastatic potential in epithelial ovarian cancer. Obstet Gynecol 69:396, 1987

Markman M: Intraperitoneal chemotherapy as treatment of ovarian carcinoma: Why, how, and when? Obstet Gynecol Surv 42:533, 1987

Micha JP, Kucora PR, Berman ML, et al: Malignant ovarian germ cell tumors: A review of thirty-six cases. Am J Obstet Gynecol 152:842, 1985

Munell EW: Is conservative therapy ever justified in stage I (IA) cancer of the ovary? Am J Obstet Gynecol 103:641, 1969

Niloff JM, Bast RC Jr, Schaetzl EM, et al: Predictive value of CA 125 antigen levels in second-look procedures for ovarian cancer. Am J Obstet Gynecol 151:981, 1985

Niloff JM, Knapp RC, Lavin PT, et al: The CA 125 assay as a predictor of clinical recurrence in epithelial ovarian cancer. Am J Obstet Gynecol 155:56, 1986

Norris HJ, Sirkin JH, Bensen WL: Immature (malignant) teratoma of the ovary. A clinical and pathologic study of 58 cases. Cancer 37:2359, 1976

Ozols RF, Ostchega Y, Myers CE, et al: High-dose cisplatin in hypertonic saline in refractory ovarian cancer. J Clin Oncol 3:1246, 1985

Phibbs GD, Smith JP, Stanhope CR: Analysis of sites of persistent cancer at "second-look" laparotomy in patients with ovarian cancer. Am J Obstet Gynecol 147:611, 1983

Piver MS, Lele SB, Pastner B, et al: Stage II invasive adenocarcinoma of the ovary: Results of treatment by whole abdominal irradiation plus pelvic boost versus pelvic radiation plus oral melphalan chemotherapy. Gynecol Oncol 23:168, 1986

Podratz KC, Malkasian GD Jr, Wieand HS, et al: Recurrent disease after negative second-look laparotomy in stages III and IV ovarian carcinoma. Gynecol Oncol 29:274, 1988

Romero R, Schwartz PE: Alpha fetoprotein determination in the management of endodermal sinus tumors and mixed germ cell tumors of the ovary. Am J Obstet Gynecol 141:126, 1981

Rosenshein NB, Hernandez E, Rosenblatt K: Risk factors for ovarian cancer. p. 221. In Gold E (ed): Changing Risks for Disease in Women: An Epidemiologic Approach. DC Heath, Lexington, MA, 1984

Schwartz PE: Combination chemotherapy in the management of ovarian germ cell malignancies. Obstet Gynecol 64:564, 1984

Serov SF, Scully RE, Sobin LH: International histologic classification of tumors, No. 9. Histological typing of ovarian tumors. World Health Organization, Geneva, 1973

Slayton RE, Park RC, Silverberg SG, et al: Vincristine, dactinomycin, and cyclophosphamide in the treatment of malignant germ cell tumors of the ovary—A Gynecologic Oncology Group study. A final report. Cancer 56:243, 1985

Smirz LR, Stehman FB, Ulbright TM, et al: Second-look laparotomy after chemotherapy in the management of ovarian malignancy. Am J Obstet Gynecol 152:661, 1985

Soper JT, Wilkerson RH Jr, Bandy LC, et al: Intraperitoneal chromic phosphate P 32 as salvage therapy for persistent carcinoma of the ovary after surgical restaging. Am J Obstet Gynecol 156:1153, 1987

Stern J, Buscema J, Rosenshein N, et al: Can computed tomography substitute for second-look operation in ovarian carcinoma? Gynecol Oncol 11:82, 1981

Taylor MH, DePetrillo AD, Turner AR: Vinblastine, bleomycin, and cisplatin in malignant germ cell tumors of the ovary. Cancer 56:1341, 1985

Thomas GM, Dembo AL, Hacker NF, et al: Current therapy for dysgerminoma of the ovary. Obstet Gynecol 70:268, 1987

Varia M, Rosenman J, Venkatraman S, et al: Intraperitoneal chromic phosphate therapy after second-look laparotomy for ovarian cancer. Cancer 61:919, 1988

Vergote IB, Bormer OP, Abeler VM: Evaluation of serum CA 125 levels in the monitoring of ovarian cancer. Am J Obstet Gynecol 157:88, 1987

Wijnen JA, Rosenshein NB: Surgery in ovarian cancer. Arch Surg 115:863, 1980

Williams CJ, Mead GM, Macbeth FR, et al: Cisplatin combination chemotherapy versus chlorambucil in advanced ovarian carcinoma: Mature results of a randomized trial. J Clin Oncol 3:1455, 1985

Williams SD, Birch R, Einhorn LH, et al: Treatment of disseminated germ-cell tumors with cisplatin, bleomycin and either vinblastine or etoposide. N Engl J Med 316:1435, 1987

Wu P-C, Qu J-Y, Lang J-H, et al: Lymph node metastasis of ovarian cancer: A preliminary survey of 74 cases of lymphadenectomy. Am J Obstet Gynecol 155:1103, 1986

Young RC, Decker DG, Wharton JT, et al: Staging laparotomy in early ovarian cancer. JAMA 250:3072, 1983

6

Gestational Trophoblastic Neoplasia

Gestational trophoblastic neoplasia (GTN) is a spectrum of disease that originates in the developing trophoblasts of pregnancy. GTN includes hydatidiform mole (complete mole), partial mole (incomplete mole), persistent mole, invasive mole, and choriocarcinoma. GTN is associated with the secretion of human chorionic gonadotropin (hCG), produced in proportion to the number of viable tumor cells. GTN is categorized and managed on the basis of extent of disease, hCG titer, duration of disease, and prior chemotherapy (Tables 6-1 and 6-2). To ensure appropriate treatment and follow-up, careful staging of the extent of disease and accurate histopathologic diagnosis is mandatory.

HISTOPATHOLOGY

Gestational trophoblastic neoplasia includes the following histopathologic entities: hydatidiform mole, invasive mole, and choriocarcinoma.

HYDATIDIFORM MOLE

The normal placenta is composed of villi and trophoblast. In hydatidiform moles there is trophoblastic proliferation, the villi are edematous (hydropic degeneration), and fetal blood vessels are typically not seen in the mesenchyme (Fig. 6-1). The hydropic degeneration of individual villi gives hydatidiform moles the appearance of a cluster of grapes, on gross examination (Fig. 6-2).

Eighty-five percent of hydatidiform moles originate from the union of an X-bearing sperm with an egg that is devoid of chromosomal material. Duplication of the sperm chromosomes results

TABLE 6-1. CLASSIFICATION OF GESTATIONAL
TROPHOBLASTIC NEOPLASIA

I. Benign GTN
    A. Hydatidiform mole (complete mole)
    B. Partial mole (incomplete mole)
II. Malignant GTN
    A. Nonmetastatic
        1. Persistent hydatidiform mole
        2. Invasive mole (chorioadenoma destruens)
        3. Choriocarcinoma
    B. Metastatic GTN
        1. Good prognosis, low-risk
            a. Serum β-hCG titer prior to therapy of less than 40,000 mIU/ml
            b. Symptoms for 4 months or less
            c. No liver or brain metastasis
            d. No previous chemotherapy
        2. Poor prognosis, high-risk
            a. Serum β-hCG titer prior to therapy of more than 40,000 mIU/ml
            b. Symptoms for more than 4 months
            c. Liver or brain metastasis
            d. Previous chemotherapy
            e. Disease following term pregnancy

in a 46XX mole, all genetic material being androgenic in origin. The other 15% of hydatidiform moles are 46XY. They result when two sperms (X- and Y-bearing) fertilize an "empty egg."

In 80% of patients with hydatidiform mole, the serum β-hCG is undetectable by 12 weeks after evacuation. In the other 20%, the serum β-hCG titers plateau or rise during follow-up. These patients are diagnosed as having malignant (or persistent) mole and should undergo metastatic evaluation and treatment with chemo-therapeutic agents (see the section *Evaluation and Management of the Patient with Malignant GTN*).

The occurrence of molar tissue with a coexisting fetus is re-fered to as partial mole. Histopathologically, partial moles are char-acterized by (1) chorionic villi with focal hydropic degeneration and cavitation, (2) focal mild to moderate trophoblastic proliferation, (3) scalloping of the chorionic villi and stromal trophoblastic inclusions, and (4) identifiable fetal or embryonic structures. The karyotype of most partial moles is 69XXY. Their clinical charac-

TABLE 6-2. WORLD HEALTH ORGANIZATION GESTATIONAL TROPHOBLASTIC NEOPLASIA PROGNOSTIC SCORING SYSTEM

Prognostic Factor	Score[a]			
	0	1	2	4
Age (years)	<39	>39	—	—
Antecedent pregnancy	Mole	Abortion	Term	
Interval (months) between end of antecedent pregnancy and start of chemotherapy	<4	4–6	7–12	>12
hCG (mIU/ml)	$<10^3$	10^3–10^4	10^4–10^5	$>10^5$
ABO groups (female × male)	—	O × A A × O	B AB	—
Largest tumor, including uterine	—	3–5 cm	>5 cm	—
Site of metastasis	—	Spleen Kidney	GI tract Liver	Brain
No. of metastases	—	1–4	4–8	>8
Prior chemotherapy	—	—	Single drug	2 or more drugs

[a] Total score: Low risk = 0–4; medium risk = 5–7; High risk = 8 or higher.
(From Bagshawe, 1984, with permission.)

teristics and natural history are not entirely dissimilar from the complete mole. The partial mole has been considered a less virulent form of molar pregnancy. Nonetheless, malignant sequelae have been reported in 4–14% of cases. Close monitoring of the serum β-hCG titers is necessary after evacuation of a partial mole.

INVASIVE MOLE (CHORIOADENOMA DESTRUENS)

A hydatidiform mole that invades deep in the myometrium or metastasizes is known as invasive mole. Invasive moles comprise about 15% of molar pregnancies in the United States. While hy-

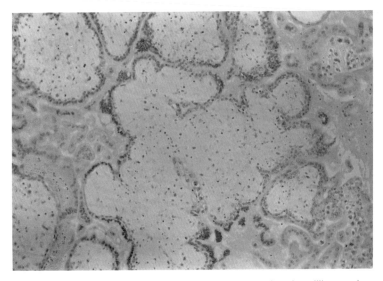

FIG. 6-1. Microscopic findings in hydatidiform mole. The villi are edematous with marked variation in size. No fetal blood vessels are identified in the mesenchyme of the villi. Trophoblastic proliferation is seen all around the villi.

datidiform mole in the United States occurs in 1 of every 1,200 pregnancies, one invasive mole occurs for every 15,000 pregnancies.

CHORIOCARCINOMA

Choriocarcinoma is histologically characterized by abundant proliferation of cytotrophoblast and syncytiotrophoblast, absence of chorionic villi, and extensive tissue necrosis and hemorrhage.

The propensity for multiple organ metastases is responsible for the varied presentations of choriocarcinoma mimicking many surgical and medical conditions. The lung is the most frequent site of metastasis, followed by lower genital tract, brain, liver, kidneys, small intestine, and spleen (Fig. 6-3).

Gestational choriocarcinoma is preceded by molar pregnancy

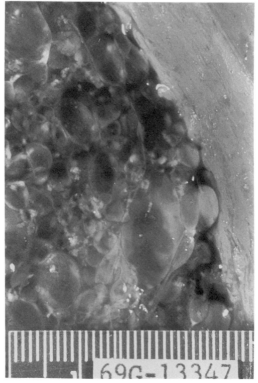

FIG. 6-2. Gross appearance of a hydatidiform mole with a mass of translucent vesicles that give the appearance of a bunch of grapes.

in 50% of cases, spontaneous abortion in 25%, normal term delivery in 22%, and an ectopic pregnancy in 3%.

EVALUATION AND MANAGEMENT OF THE PATIENT WITH BENIGN GTN

WORKUP

1. Hemoglobin
2. Hepatorenal profile
3. Coagulation studies, including prothrombin time (PT) and partial thromboplastin time (PTT)

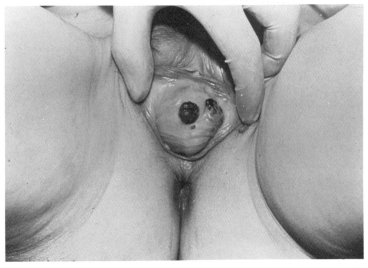

FIG. 6-3. Choriocarcinoma metastatic to the lower genital tract. This lesion can bleed profusely if biopsied.

4. Serum β-hCG
5. Free thyroxine (T_4)
6. Type and hold for 2 U of packed red blood cells (PRBC)
7. Urinalysis
8. Chest radiographs, both posteroanterior (PA) and lateral
9. Pelvic ultrasound
10. Electrocardiogram (ECG) if indicated by age (45 or older), or clinical findings

TREATMENT

1. Suction and sharp dilatation and curettage (D & C), or consider hysterectomy if childbearing completed
2. Careful fluid and electrolyte management
3. Histologic confirmation of diagnosis
4. Postoperative chest radiographs if signs and/or symptoms of pulmonary edema develop
5. Administration of Rhogam if Rh negative

FOLLOW-UP

1. Weekly serum β-hCG until four normal values are obtained, then once a month for a year; if the β-hCG titer declines but is still detectable at 16 weeks after D & C, reevaluation is indicated
2. Physical examination 4, 8, and 12 weeks after D & C, then every 3 months for 1 year
3. Contraception during the follow-up period (e.g., 1 year of undetectable serum β-hCG); oral contraceptives preferred
4. Possibility of intrauterine pregnancy during the year of follow-up—should be confirmed with pelvic ultrasound
5. Subsequent pregnancies—require early sonographic confirmation

Plateauing or rising titers require workup and staging for malignant/metastatic disease.

EVALUATION AND MANAGEMENT OF THE PATIENT WITH MALIGNANT GTN

WORKUP

1. Hemogram (CBC)
2. Hepatorenal profile: electrolytes, blood urea nitrogen (BUN), glucose, creatinine, bilirubin, transaminases, lactate dehydrogenase (LDH), protein, uric acid, cholesterol, alkaline phosphatase, calcium, phosphorus
3. Coagulation studies: PT, PTT
4. Serum β-hCG
5. Free T_4
6. Blood type and Rh
7. Urinalysis
8. Cervical cytology
9. Chest radiographs: PA and lateral; CT if indicated
10. Abdominal/pelvic CT
11. CT of the head
12. ECG if indicated by age (45 or older), or clinical findings
13. Medical consultation as indicated
14. Additional studies if indicated
    a. Electroencephalogram (EEG)

    b. Selected arteriography
    c. Cerebrospinal fluid (CSF) hCG level
15. Presentation to the Gynecologic Oncology Tumor Board when workup completed

TREATMENT AND FOLLOW-UP

Malignant GTN, Nonmetastatic

1. Single-agent chemotherapy with methotrexate or actinomycin-D for 5 days every 3 weeks (see specific chemotherapy protocols, Ch. 7)
2. D & C or total abdominal hysterectomy on third day of first course of treatment
3. Treatment continues for one course following a normal serum β-hCG titer.
4. Serum β-hCG every week, until four negative titers are obtained, then every month for 12 months.
5. Contraception for 1 year. Oral contraceptives are preferred.
6. If serum β-hCG titers plateau or rise, alternate drug should be used; failure of alternate drug or development of metastasis requires multi-agent chemotherapy

Malignant GTN, Metastatic

1. Good-prognosis metastatic GTN treated as nonmetastatic GTN
2. Poor-prognosis metastatic GTN
    a. Chemotherapy (see Ch. 7)
       Primary regimen
          Methotrexate–actinomycin–cyclophosphamide (MAC)
       Secondary regimens
          Bleomycin–etoposide–*cis*-platinum (BEP)
          Etoposide–methotrexate–actinomycin/cyclophosphamide–vincristine (EMA/CO)
          Einhorn regimen (*cis*-platinum–vinblastine–bleomycin)
          Modified Bagshawe regimen (hydroxyurea–vincristine–methotrexate–actinomycin-D–cyclophosphamide–Adriamycin–folinic acid)
    b. Whole-brain irradiation (3,000 cGy) for documented brain metastasis: dexamethasone (e.g., Decadron), 4 mg twice to four times a day to reduce brain edema
    c. Liver irradiation (2,000 cGy) for documented hepatic metastasis; consider hepatic arterial embolization to control bleeding

d. Treatment continued until two courses past a normal serum β-hCG titer
e. Serum β-hCG every week until four negative titers obtained, then every month for 12 months
f. Contraception for 1 year; oral contraceptives preferred
g. Choriocarcinoma can recur after several years in remission: follow-up serum β-hCG titers obtained every 3 months during the second year, and every 6 months thereafter
h. Subsequent pregnancies—require early sonographic evaluation

SUGGESTED READINGS

Amir SM, Osathanondh R, Berkowitz RS: Human chorionic gonadotropin and thyroid function in patients with hydatidiform mole. Am J Obstet Gynecol 150:723, 1984

Atrash HK, Hogue CJR, Grimes DA: Epidemiology of hydatidiform mole during early gestation. Am J Obstet Gynecol 154:906, 1986

Bagshawe KD: Risk and prognostic factors in trophoblastic neoplasm. Cancer 38:1373, 1976

Bagshawe KD: Treatment of high-risk choriocarcinoma. J Reprod Med 29:813, 1984

Barnard DE, Woodward KT, Yancy SG, et al: Hepatic metastases of choriocarcinoma: A report of 15 patients. Gynecol Oncol 25:73, 1986

DuBeshter B, Berkowitz RS, Goldstein DP et al: Metastatic gestational trophoblastic disease: Experience at the New England Trophoblastic Disease Center 1965 to 1985. Obstet Gynecol 69:390, 1987

Galton VA, Ingbar SH, Jimenez-Fonseca J, et al: Alterations in thyroid hormone economy in patients with hydatidiform mole. J Clin Invest 50:1345, 1971

Gordon AN, Gershenson DM, Copeland LJ, et al: High-risk metastatic gestational trophoblastic disease. Obstet Gynecol 65:550, 1985

Gordon AN, Kavanagh JJ, Gershenson DM, et al: Cisplatin, vinblastine, and bleomycin combination therapy in resistant gestational trophoblastic disease. Cancer 58:1407, 1986

Grimes DA: Epidemiology of gestational trophoblastic disease. Am J Obstet Gynecol 150:309, 1984

Grumbine FC, Rosenshein NB, Brereton HD, et al: Management of liver metastasis from gestational trophoblastic neoplasia. Am J Obstet Gynecol 137:959, 1980

Hammond CB, Borchert LG, Tyrey L, et al: Treatment of metastatic trophoblastic disease. Good and poor prognosis. Am J Obstet Gynecol 115:451, 1973

Hammond CB, Weed JC Jr, Currie JL: The role of operation in the current therapy of gestational trophoblastic disease. Am J Obstet Gynecol 136:844, 1980

Ilancheran A, Ratnam SS, Baratham G: Metastatic cerebral choriocarcinoma with primary neurological presentation. Gynecol Oncol 29:361, 1988

Kajii T, Ohama K: Androgenetic origin of hydatidiform mole. Nature (Lond) 268:633, 1977

McDonald TW, Ruffolo EH: Modern management of gestational trophoblastic disease. Obstet Gynecol Surv 38:67, 1983

Morrow P, Nakamura R, Schlaerth J, et al: The influence of oral contraceptives on the postmolar human chorionic gonadotropin regression curve. Am J Obstet Gynecol 151:906, 1985

Newlands ES: VP-16 in combinations for first-time treatment of malignant germ-cell tumors and gestational choriocarcinoma. Semin Oncol 12 (suppl 2):37, 1985

Newlands ES, Rustin GJS, Bagshawe KD, et al: Weekly EMA/CO chemotherapy for high-risk gestational trophoblastic tumors. Proc American Society of Clinical Oncology 5:112, 1986 (abst)

Rotmensch J, Rosenshein NB, Block BS: Comparison of human chorionic gonadotropin regression in molar pregnancies and post-molar nonmetastatic gestational trophoblastic neoplasia. Gynecol Oncol 29:82, 1988

Sand PK, Lurain JR, Brewer JI: Repeat gestational trophoblastic disease. Obstet Gynecol 63:140, 1984

Song H, Wu, P, Wang Y, et al: Pregnancy outcome after successful chemotherapy for choriocarcinoma and invasive mole: Long-term follow-up. Am J Obstet Gynecol 158:538, 1988

Surwit EA: The management of poor prognosis trophoblastic disease. Semin Oncol 9:204, 1982

Surwit EA, Alberts DS, Christian CD: Poor-prognosis gestational trophoblastic disease: An update. Obstet Gynecol 64:21, 1984

Twiggs LB, Morrow CP, Schlaerth JB: Acute pulmonary complications of molar pregnancy. Am J Obstet Gynecol 135:189, 1979

Vejerslev LO, Dueholm M, Nielsen FH: Hydatidiform mole: Cytogenetic marker analysis in twin gestation. Am J Obstet Gynecol 155:614, 1986

Vejerslev LO, Fisher RA, Surti U, et al: Hydatidiform mole: cytogenetically unusual cases and their implications for the present classification. Am J Obstet Gynecol 157:180, 1987

Wahl RL, Khazaeli MB, LoBuglio AF, et al: Radioimmunoscintigraphic detection of occult gestational choriocarcinoma. Am J Obstet Gynecol 156:108, 1987

Watson EJ, Hernandez E, Miyazawa K: Partial hydatidiform moles: A review. Obstet Gynecol Surv 42:540, 1987

Weed JC Jr, Barnard DE, Currie JL, et al: Chemotherapy with the modified Bagshawe protocol for poor prognosis metastatic trophoblastic disease. Obstet Gynecol 59:377, 1982

Weed JC Jr, Hammond CB: Cerebral metastatic choriocarcinoma: Intensive therapy and prognosis. Obstet Gynecol 55:89, 1980

Yordan EL Jr, Schlaerth J, Gaddis O, et al: Radiation therapy in the management of gestational choriocarcinoma metastatic to the central nervous system. Obstet Gynecol 69:627, 1987

Yuen BH, Cannon W: Molar pregnancy in British Columbia: Estimated incidence and postevacuation regression patterns of the beta subunit of human chorionic gonadotropin. Am J Obstet Gynecol 139:316, 1981

7

Chemotherapy

Chemotherapy is administered as adjuvant therapy to eradicate micrometastases, as neoadjuvant therapy to reduce tumor volume before surgery or radiation, and as therapy for disseminated or recurrent cancer. Some gynecologic malignancies are treated primarily with chemotherapy. The major aim of chemotherapy is to produce maximum cancer cell kill with minimum toxicity. Dosage schedules for administration are designed in an effort to achieve this end.

GENERAL GUIDELINES

1. A short Silastic catheter (e.g., Angiocath) is used for intravenous (IV) access.
2. A hemogram and platelet count should be done within 24 hours of administration of chemotherapy.
   a. The white blood cell (WBC) count must be greater than 3,000 mm^3 for full dose of bone marrow depressant drugs. (A 25% dose reduction is made if the nadir WBC count was less than 1,500 mm^3.)
   b. Platelets must be greater than 100,000 mm^3 for full dose of bone marrow depressant drugs. (A 25% dose reduction is made if the nadir platelet count was less than 50,000 mm^3.)
   c. All patients must have a hematocrit above 25% before they are discharged.
3. A current electrocardiogram (ECG) must be on the chart when a patient is receiving a cardiotoxic drug (e.g., Adriamycin). Baseline and serial left ventricular ejection fractions should be obtained in patients with cardiac risk factors who are receiving Adriamycin.
4. Baseline and periodic pulmonary function studies are obtained for patients receiving a pulmonary toxic drug (e.g., bleomycin).
5. A chemotherapy flow sheet should be kept. This flow sheet should summarize the drugs, doses, and dates of administration.

6. When the patient is receiving a drug causing nausea and vomiting, an antiemetic is administered 30 minutes before the onset of treatment (see the section *Antiemetics, antiemetic protocol*).

7. When the patient is receiving a renal/bladder toxic agent, she is hydrated before and after treatment (e.g., 3–4 L/day intravenously or orally, according to protocol).

8. When the patient is receiving a bladder toxic agent (e.g., Cytoxan), encourage frequent voiding.

9. A recent serum creatinine and/or creatinine clearance must be on the chart when a patient is receiving a nephrotoxic drug (e.g., methotrexate, *cis*-platinum). Appropriate reduction in chemotherapeutic agents excreted mainly by the kidney must be made if renal impairment is found.

10. If a vesicant drug is being administered (e.g., Adriamycin, actinomycin D, vincristine), the house officer must be in attendance throughout the infusion to be certain that the infusion is definitely INTRAVENOUS.

11. If a vesicant drug infiltrates, STOP the infusion, and try to aspirate back. If it is an anthracene (e.g., Adriamycin) or antibiotic (e.g., actinomycin), ice should be applied intermittently for the first 24 hours. If a vinca alkaloid (e.g., vincristine), inject 150 U of hyaluronidase in 2 ml of normal saline at the site of infiltration. Apply moist warm packs.

12. If the granulocyte count falls below 1,000 mm^3, infection prevention measures should be initiated:
    a. Protective isolation
    b. Observation for infection, especially respiratory, urinary, perineal, and IV access site
    c. No enemas
    d. If temperature rises above 38.3°C—appropriate cultures should be taken and the patient should be started on appropriate antibiotics

13. If platelets fall below 40,000 mm^3, bleeding prevention measures should be initiated:
    a. No IM or subcutaneous (SC) injections
    b. No rectal temperatures
    c. No enemas or douches
    d. Observation for hemorrhage, especially at IV access sites, old injection sites, joints, and mucous membranes

14. All chemotherapy should be written in the following format:
    Height   Weight   Body Surface Area
    Dosage of drug to be given according to protocol
    Patient's calculated dosage

    EXAMPLE:
    Height 64 inches   Weight 120 pounds   BSA 1.57 m^2
    cis-platinum 50 mg/m^2
    Give *cis*-platinum 78.5 mg

ANTIEMETICS

GENERAL GUIDELINES

Nausea and vomiting is a frequent side effect of antineoplastic agents. The use of antiemetics provides patient comfort and increases compliance.

1. Always pretreat the patient (e.g., start antiemetics 30 minutes before chemotherapy administration).
2. Do not use a prn (as needed) dosing schedule for the first 24 hours after chemotherapy administration.
3. Use combinations of agents from the different classes of antiemetics.
4. Be aggressive in pushing the doses of these agents. The goal is to stop the nausea and vomiting. The side effects of the antiemetics can be treated.

Table 7-1 depicts a list of frequently used antiemetics, their dosages and possible side effects.

ANTIEMETIC PROTOCOL

1. Patients receiving a chemotherapy regimen that includes *cis*-platinum can receive the following antiemetic protocol if no contraindications to the use of the individual drugs are present.
   a. Metoclopromide (Reglan), 2 mg/kg in 100 ml of 5% dextrose given IV over 15 minutes, 30 minutes before chemotherapy, and again 1.5, 3.5, 6.5, 9.5, and 12.5 hours after initiation of chemotherapy

TABLE 7-1. GUIDE TO ANTIEMETICS USED IN THE MANAGEMENT OF CHEMOTHERAPY-INDUCED NAUSEA AND VOMITING

Drug	Starting Dose	Route of Administration	Adverse Effects	Comments
Prochlorperazine (e.g., Compazine)	10 mg q6h 25 mg q6h 5–10 mg q6h	Oral (PO) Rectal (PR) Intramuscular (IM)	Extrapyramidal symptoms (EPS): tardive dyskinesias Sedation Dry mouth	Benadryl, 50 mg q6h will prevent EPS and aid as an antiemetic
Chloropromazine (e.g., Thorazine)	25–50 mg q6h	Oral Rectal Intramuscular	Tachycardia Nausea and vomiting Syndrome of inappropriate anti-diuretic hormone secretion Gynecomastia	
Droperidol (e.g., Inapsine)	5–15 mg IV push, then 1.25–3 mg/hr continuous infusion 1.25–2.5 mg q2–3h	Intravenous (IV) Intramuscular		
Haloperidol (e.g., Haldol)	1–2 mg q6h	Oral Rectal Intramuscular		

Drug	Dose	Route	Side Effects	Comments
Metoclopromide (e.g., Reglan)	1–3 mg/kg q2h for 3 doses, then q3h for 2 doses	Oral Intravenous	As above plus: diarrhea, nausea, and vomiting; urinary retention	Treat diarrhea with Lomotil, Imodium, or Paregoric
Dexamethasone (e.g., Decadron)	20 mg IV push 30 min prior to chemotherapy, then 10 mg PO q6h	Oral Intramuscular Intravenous	Sodium and water retention Immunosuppression Nausea and vomiting	Useful as an adjunct; not recommended as a single agent
Diphenhydramine (e.g., Benadryl)	50 mg q6h	Oral Intramuscular Intravenous	Dry mouth Nausea and vomiting Sedation Urinary retention	Not effective as a single agent Very useful in combination with other agents Antidote for EPS
Hydroxyzine (e.g., Vistaril)	50–100 mg qid	Oral Intramuscular	CNS depression Sedation Dry mouth	Not effective as a single agent
Diazepam (e.g., Valium)	2–10 mg bid to qid	Oral Intravenous Intramuscular	Sedation; CNS depression Diarrhea Constipation Nausea and vomiting	Useful when nausea and vomiting have an anxiety component
Lorazepam (e.g., Ativan)	1–2 mg tid	Oral Intramuscular Intravenous	—	—

    b. Diphenhydramine (Benadryl), 50 mg IM 30 min before chemotherapy and every 6 hours for at least 4 doses

    c. Dexamethasone (Decadron), 20 mg by IV push 30 minutes before chemotherapy, followed by 10 mg PO every 6 hours for 4 doses (Do not use in patients with severe diabetes, active tuberculosis, cataracts, glaucoma, peptic ulcer, psychiatric problems.)

2. Patients on chemotherapy regimens of more than 1 day do not receive Decadron. Lorazepam (Ativan), 1 mg can be given three times a day by the PO, IM, or IV route.

3. Other agents recommended for the patient that cannot receive the above are:

    a. Chlorpromazine (Thorazine), 50 mg IM every 4 hours

    b. Droperidol (Inapsine), 5–15 mg by IV push, followed by 1.5–3 mg/hr continuous infusion or 1.25–2.5 mg IM every 2–3 hours

4. Note in the chart the effectiveness of the antiemetic regimen used (e.g., number of episodes of nausea and vomiting, and severity) and side effects (e.g., extrapyramidal symptoms, diarrhea, electrolyte imbalance).

CHEMOTHERAPEUTIC AGENTS

A list of chemotherapeutic agents used for the treatment of gynecologic malignancies is presented in Table 7-2.

MULTIPLE DRUG CHEMOTHERAPY

Combination chemotherapy is administered in an effort to enhance the cancer cell killing ability of individual drugs. The individual drugs used in polychemotherapy regimens are known to be active against the malignancy being treated. They should have different mechanisms of action and should produce toxicities that occur in different organ systems and at different times after their administration. These regimens should be used in repeated brief courses in order to minimize the immunosuppressive effects that might otherwise occur.

MULTIPLE DRUG THERAPY PROTOCOLS

The side effects and comments on management are the same as for the individual drugs, as previously outlined (see Table 7-2). Methods of administration and procedures are the same unless otherwise indicated.

MAC

Methotrexate 0.3 mg/kg IV (max 15 mg)

Actinomycin D 0.01 mg/kg IV (max 0.5 mg)

Cyclophosphamide (Cytoxan) 3–5 mg/kg IV (max 250 mg)

Administer daily for 5 days and repeat every 2–3 weeks.

Indications: High-risk gestational trophoblastic neoplasia, ovarian choriocarcinoma

Side Effects: Bone marrow depression, potentially severe gastrointestinal (GI) toxicity (nausea, stomatitis, diarrhea)
Alopecia
Hemorrhagic cystitis (secondary to Cytoxan metabolites)
Phlebitis, local ulceration (secondary to actinomycin D)

Comments on Management: Monitor intake and output.
Administer actinomycin in free-flowing IV—STOP if infiltration occurs.
Provide oral hygiene.
Check hemogram and platelets.
Hydrate to prevent hemorrhagic cystitis that can be caused by Cytoxan.
Encourage frequent voidings.

VAC

Vincristine 1.5 mg/m^2 IV (max 2 mg)	Day 1
Actinomycin D 0.01 mg/kg IV (max 0.5 mg)	Day 1–5
Cytoxan 5 mg/kg IV (max 250 mg)	Day 1–5

Treatment is repeated every 4 weeks.

Indications: Sarcomas, malignant germ cell tumors

(*Text continues on page 100.*)

TABLE 7-2. CHEMOTHERAPEUTIC AGENTS USED FOR MECHANISMS OF ACTION, ROUTE OF ADMINISTRATION,

Agent	Route	Indications
Alkylating agents: Crosslinks DNA nucleotides interfering with DNA replications and RNA		
Cyclophosphamide Cytoxan (CTX)—cycle specific, phase nonspecific	IV (PO)	Ovarian cancer Uterine sarcoma Cervical cancer Malignant germ cell tumors Endometrial cancer
Melphalan Phenylalanine mustard Alkeran L-Pam—cycle specific, phase nonspecific	PO (IV)	Ovarian carcinoma
Chlorambucil Leukeran—cycle specific	PO	Ovarian adenocarcinoma Choriocarcinoma Malignant germ cell tumors
Antimetabolites: Similar in structure to normal metabolites; interferes with synthesis of		
Methotrexate (MTX)—phase specific (S phase) Folic acid antagonist: binds dihydrofolate reductase, preventing pyrimidine synthesis	IM IV PO Intrathecally	Malignant trophoblastic disease Cervical carcinoma Malignant germ cell tumors
Fluorouracil 5-FU—phase-specific (S phase) Pyrimidine analogue: inhibits thymidylate synthetase thus inhibiting DNA synthesis	IV Topical	Ovarian carcinoma Metastatic endometrial cancer Cervical cancer Malignant gestational trophoblastic neoplasia Vaginal and vulvar condyloma and intraepithelial neoplasia
Mercaptopurine 6-MP—phase specific (S phase) Purine antagonist	PO	Trophoblastic disease

THE TREATMENT OF GYNECOLOGIC MALIGNANCIES: INDICATIONS, ACUTE AND DELAYED SIDE EFFECTS

Acute Side Effects	Delayed Side Effects	Comments
transcription and protein synthesis, resulting in the death of the cell		
Nausea, vomiting	Bone marrow depression 7–14 days after dose Platelet sparing Alopecia Liver dysfunction Hemorrhagic cystitis	Force fluids = hydrate 3 L/day, IV or PO. Encourage frequent voidings. Monitor intake and output. Check hemogram and platelets. Medicate for nausea.
Mild nausea	Bone marrow depression (especially platelets)	Check platelets. Give after meals.
Rare: nausea and vomiting Diarrhea	Bone marrow depression with prolonged high dose Hepatotoxicity Dermatitis	Check hemogram and platelets.
DNA, RNA, and certain enzymes		
Nausea, vomiting Diarrhea High-dose—*Acute renal failure*	Oral and GI ulcerations Bone marrow depression Hepatic toxicity Renal toxicity	Hydrate (3 L/day). Strict monitoring of intake and output. Check renal function. Provide oral hygiene. Check for tarry stools, hematemesis. Check hemogram and platelets. Check other medications: effect of MTX decreased by simultaneous use of weak organic acids such as salicylates, sulfonamides, and aminobenzoic acid. Also sulfonamides displace MTX from plasma protein-binding sites, increasing MTX toxicity.
Nausea, vomiting Diarrhea Anorexia	Oral and GI ulcerations Bone marrow depression Alopecia Nail changes Dermatitis Increase pigmentation, toughening of skin Cerebellar ataxia (rare)	Provide oral hygiene. Check for tarry stools. Medicate for nausea, diarrhea. Check hemogram and platelets. Decrease dose if kidney or liver function impaired. High risk in presence of infection.
Nausea, vomiting Diarrhea Stomatitis	Bone marrow depression Liver dysfunction	Check dose: if patient taking allopurinol for hyperuricemia, 6 MP should be decreased to no more than one-third of usual dose, since allopurinol delays its metabolism and increases its potency. Check hemogram and platelets.

(continued)

TABLE 7-2.

Agent	Route	Indications
Antibiotics: Inhibit DNA and/or RNA synthesis.		

Dactinomycin
    Actinomycin D (cycle specific)
    Binds with enzyme to block
    DNA-dependent RNA
    synthesis to cause cell injury
    and death.
	IV (vesicant)	Gestational trophoblastic
		    disease
		Epithelial ovarian carcinoma
		Uterine sarcoma
		Malignant germ cell tumors

Bleomycin
    Blenoxane (maximal action in S
    phase)
    Binds directly to DNA causing
    strand scission and resulting
    in reduced synthesis of DNA,
    RNA, and proteins
	IM
	IV
		Epithelial tumors: squamous
		    cell carcinoma of cervix,
		    vagina, vulva
		Malignant germ cell tumors

Doxorubicin
    Adriamycin (maximal action in
    S phase)
    Inhibits nucleic acid synthesis
	IV (vesicant)	Ovarian carcinoma
		Sarcomas
		Endometrial cancer
		Gestational trophoblastic
		    neoplasia

Mitomycin C
    Mutamycin
        Crosslinks DNA, inhibits
        DNA synthesis, and breaks
        down RNA
	IV (vesicant)	Cervical carcinoma

continued

Acute Side Effects	Delayed Side Effects	Comments
Vesicant—nausea, vomiting Diarrhea Phlebitis Anorexia	Oral and GI ulcerations Alopecia Bone marrow depression 1–7 days after dose Gastrointestinal symptoms worse with radiation therapy	Administer through a free-flowing IV infusion. Check IV site. Provide oral hygiene (hydrogen peroxide rinse). Check hemogram and platelets. Stop infusion. If infiltrates, apply ice. Administer antiemetics.
Occasional vomiting, nausea Fever Shocklike syndrome Hypotension Pulmonary edema Anaphylaxis	Pneumonitis—fibrosis Alopecia, nail changes, skin ulcerations Anorexia	Monitor vital signs every 15 minutes during initial infusion. Caution if renal or pulmonary disease. TOTAL DOSE NOT TO EXCEED 200 mg/m^2. Stop if DL_{CO} less than 50% or if drops more than 20%. If anorexia present, encourage small frequent feedings.
Vesicant—Severe tissue damage if infiltrates Nausea, vomiting, diarrhea Red urine (not hematuria)	Bone marrow depression Cardiotoxicity (incidence of congestive heart failure increases exponentially with doses over 550 mg/m^2). Alopecia Gastrointestinal ulcerations. Hepatic damage Skin burning, erythema, that can progress to ulceration and necrosis. Radiation recall.	Administer through a free-flowing IV infusion. Stop infusion immediately if infiltrates, apply ice. If cardiac disease, obtain ejection fraction (e.g., MUGA scan). Obtain ECG prior to each dose. Check hemogram and platelets. Decrease dose with impaired liver function. Toxicity increases in elderly. Total cumulative dose not to exceed 550 mg/m^2. Stop if ejection fraction less than 45%.
Vesicant—local reaction if extravasates Nausea, vomiting Fever	Bone marrow depression (cumulative) Renal toxicity Alopecia Stomatitis	Administer through a free-flowing IV infusion.

(continued)

TABLE 7-2.

Agent	Route	Indications
Antibiotics (*continued*)		
Mithramycin Mithracin Inhibits RNA synthesis	IV	Hypercalcemia
Vinca alkaloids: Mitosis-arresting drugs		
Vincristine Oncovin [phase-specific (mitosis)]	IV (vesicant)	Cervical squamous cell carcinoma Endometrial sarcoma Malignant germ cell tumors
Vinblastine Velban [phase specific (mitosis)]	IV (vesicant)	Choriocarcinoma Malignant germ cell tumors
Miscellaneous drugs		
Cis-platinum Platinol Heavy metal Crosslinks DNA, preventing DNA synthesis	IV	Ovarian carcinoma Cervical carcinoma Malignant germ cell tumors Gestational trophoblastic neoplasia

continued

Acute Side Effects	Delayed Side Effects	Comments
Nausea, vomiting Diarrhea	Hemorrhagic diathesis Bone marrow depression Liver, renal toxicities Hypocalcemia Hypokalemia Stomatitis Headaches, drowsiness, depression	VERY TOXIC DRUG Check LDH, BUN, prothrombin time (PT), hemogram and platelets before each dose. Contraindicated in patients with kidney/liver dysfunction, coagulation disorders. Strictly monitor intake and output. Observe for signs and symptoms of bleeding; check stool guaiac (e.g., Hemoccult). Medicate for nausea, vomiting, and diarrhea.
Vesicant: severe local reaction	Dose-related alopecia Neurotoxic: peripheral neuropathy, paresthesia, loss of deep tendon reflexes, unsteady gait, loss of coordination, constipation paralytic ileus, areflexias, abdominal and mandibular pain Occasional bone marrow depression.	Administer through a free-flowing IV infusion. Stop infusion immediately if infiltrates. Question dose if reflexes are depressed or paresthesias are present. Prophylactic cathartics may be indicated. Check hemogram and platelets. MAXIMUM DOSE AT ANY ONE TIME IS 2 mg.
Vesicant—nausea, vomiting	Bone marrow depression (leukopenia is dose limiting) Alopecia Malaise, paresthesias Phlebitis Anorexia	Check hemogram. Check IV site, STOP if infiltrates. If anorexia present, encourage small frequent feedings. Check for constipation and urinary retention.
Severe nausea, vomiting Tinnitus	Progressive renal failure (reabsorption in distal tubules) Bone marrow depression 12–16 days after dose Hearing deficit at higher frequencies	Check hemogram and platelets. Check serum creatinine: if greater than 1.5, obtain creatinine clearance. Hydrate: 1000 ml NS with 20 mEq/L KCl over 6 hr prior to *cis*-platinum. Continue infusion for 8 hr after *cis*-platinum or until patient is able to tolerate oral fluids.

(*continued*)

TABLE 7-2.

Agent	Route	Indications
Miscellaneous drugs (*continued*)		
Cis-platinum (*continued*)		

VP-16
  Etoposide
  VePesid (phase-specific-G2,
    DNA synthesis inhibition,
    metaphase arrest)
	IV	Malignant germ cell tumors
		Gestational trophoblastic
		  neoplasia

Dacarbazine
  DTIC
  Thought to act by crosslinking
    of DNA
	IV (vesicant)	Malignant melanoma
		Uterine sarcoma

Hydroxyurea
  Hydrea
  May act as DNA-selective
    antimetabolite by interfering
    with the enzymatic
    conversion of ribonucleotides
    to deoxyribonucleotides.
  May directly damage DNA by
    inhibiting incorporation of
    thymidine into DNA.
	PO	

Side Effects: Bone marrow depression
Hemorrhagic cystitis
Neurotoxicity
Gastrointestinal toxicity
Alopecia
Phlebitis, local ulceration

Comments on
Management: Administer in free flowing IV—STOP if infiltration occurs.
Monitor intake and output.
Provide oral hygiene.
Administer antiemetics.

continued

Acute Side Effects	Delayed Side Effects	Comments
	Neuropathies (dose related)	Administer antiemetics ½ hour prior to infusion and after *cis*-platinum as per antiemetic protocol; concurrent infusion of diuretic as per protocol for doses greater than 75 mg/m^2. Urinary output should be greater than 200 ml/hr for doses over 75 mg/m^2.
Nausea, vomiting (30%) Hypotension (1%) Anaphylactic reaction (1–2%)	Myelosuppression WBC nadir days 7–14 Platelets nadir days 9–16 Anorexia (10%) Stomatitis (1%) Diarrhea (1–13%) Alopecia (8–20%) Peripheral neuropathy (1–3%)	Administer in 500 ml normal saline over 1 hour. Do not give by rapid IV push. Administer antiemetics. Watch and be ready to treat anaphylactic reaction. Get hemogram 10–14 days after treatment.
Vesicant—nausea, vomiting, anorexia, flulike syndrome: myalgias, malaise, temperature to 39°C	Bone marrow depression Hepatic toxicity Alopecia	Administer in free-flowing IV infusion. STOP infusion if infiltrates and apply ice immediately. Administer antiemetics as needed. Check hemogram, platelets, liver enzymes.
Nausea, vomiting, diarrhea, or constipation	Bone marrow depression—dose related Stomatitis—rare Dysuria, azotemia Neurotoxicity is rare (e.g., headache, dizziness, disorientation)	—

Check hemogram and platelets.
Hydrate before and after Cytoxan, 3 L/day IV or PO, depending on ability to take oral fluids.
Encourage frequent voidings.

Act–Fu–Cy

Actinomycin D, 0.01 mg/kg IV

5-Fluorouracil (5-Fu), 5 mg/kg IV

Cytoxan, 5 mg/kg IV

Administer daily for 5 days and repeat every 4 weeks.

Indications: Ovarian carcinoma, malignant germ cell tumors without choriocarcinoma, malignant stromal tumors

Side Effects: Potentially severe bone marrow depression and GI toxicity (stomatitis, nausea, vomiting)
Dermatitis, tissue necrosis
Hemorrhagic cystitis
Phlebitis, local ulceration

Comments on
Management: Check hemogram and platelets.
Monitor intake and output.
Administer in free-flowing IV line—STOP infusion if infiltration occurs.
Hydrate before and after Cytoxan.
Encourage frequent voidings.
Provide oral hygiene.
Administer antiemetics.

High-Dose *Cis*-platinum

Cis-platinum 100 mg/m^2
Repeated every 4 weeks
Cis-platinum infused in 500 ml, 3% saline over 2 hours
375 ml of 10% mannitol solution infused through second IV line concurrently with *cis*-platinum

Indications: Carcinoma of the ovary, cervix, renal pelvis, ureter, bladder

Side Effects: Bone marrow depression
Ototoxicity
Nephrotoxicity
Neuropathies
Electrolyte imbalances to include hypomagnesemia

Comments on
Management: Check WBC count and platelets.
Check serum creatinine.
Obtain creatinine clearance if serum creatinine abnormal or rising.
Consider audiogram prior to first dose as a baseline; repeat if patient complains of tinnitus or hearing deficit.

Electrolytes and blood urea nitrogen (BUN) should be checked 18 hours after completion of infusion.

Strict intake and output; insert Foley catheter with urimeter.

Maintain urinary output over 200 ml/hr.

Hydration: Patient given 1,000 ml normal saline with 20 mEq/L of potassium chloride IV over 4 hours prior to *cis*-platinum. After completion of *cis*-platinum infusion—5% dextrose-0.45 NS + 20 mEq/L KCl at 125 ml/hr until able to tolerate oral fluids

Protocol for Endometrial Cancer

Megace 80 mg PO BID

Cytoxan 500 mg/m^2 IV, day 1, repeat every 4 weeks

Adriamycin 40 mg/m^2 IV, day 1, repeat every 4 weeks

Reassess after 3–4 courses; if patient has stable or progressive disease add *cis*-platinum 50 mg/m^2 IV in 500 ml of normal saline over 2 hours every 4 weeks

If estrogen receptor positive but progesterone receptor negative, Tamoxifen is used instead of Megace. The Tamoxifen dose is 20 mg BID

Indications: Metastatic and inoperable uterine carcinoma

Side Effects: Bone marrow depression
Liver toxicity
Gastrointestinal toxicity
Hemorrhagic cystitis
Stomatitis
Tissue necrosis
Cardiac toxicity
Renal toxicity

Comments on Management: Check hemogram and platelets before treatment and 2 weeks after treatment.
Check bilirubin.
Administer antiemetics.
Hydrate before and after Cytoxan—3 L/day IV or PO.
Encourage frequent voidings.
Provide oral hygiene.

Check ECG.

Check total dose of Adriamycin—must be less than 550 mg/m^2.

PAC

Cis-platinum 50 mg/m^2 in 500 ml normal saline IV over 2 hours

Adriamycin 40 mg/m^2 IV push by house officer through a wide open IV line

Cytoxan 500 mg/m^2 in 100 ml, 5% dextrose infused over 15–20 minutes

If there is a history of cardiac disease or the cardiac ejection fraction is less than 45%, do not give Adriamycin; increase Cytoxan dose to 750–1,000 mg/m^2.

Repeat every 28 days.

Indications: Ovarian carcinoma
Uterine carcinoma
Malignant gonadostromal tumors
Mixed mesordermal tumors

Side Effects: Bone marrow depression
Severe nausea and vomiting
Tissue necrosis
Hemorrhagic cystitis
Cardiomyopathy
Renal toxicity
Electrolyte imbalance
Alopecia
Ototoxicity
Peripheral neuropathy

Comments on Management: Check hemogram and platelets.
Administer in free-flowing IV—STOP if infiltration occurs.
Administer antiemetics.
Before chemotherapy infusion, hydrate by giving 1,000 ml of 0.45 normal saline + 20 mEq/L KCl IV at 150–175 ml/hr.
After this initial liter, give an additional 2 L of 0.2 NS + 20 mEq/L KCl at 125 ml/hr.
Monitor intake and output.

If urinary output is less than 50 ml/hr, an increase in the IV infusion rate and diuresis with furosemide (Lasix) or mannitol may be required.

Check total dose of Adriamycin—not to exceed 550 mg/m^2.

Check ECG (decrease in voltage, arrhythmias, ST depression, flattening or inversion of T waves).

Check for signs and symptoms of congestive heart failure.

Obtain baseline and serial left ventricular ejection fraction if indicated.

Check serum creatinine.

Obtain creatinine clearance if serum creatinine abnormal or rising.

Obtain serum electrolytes to include magnesium.

Check for neurotoxicity.

Provide oral hygiene.

Modified Einhorn (PVB)

Cis-platinum 20 mg/m^2 in 250 ml of normal saline as a 15- to 30-minute infusion, days 1–5 and repeated every 3 weeks

Vinblastine 0.15 mg/kg (6 mg/m^2) IV on days 1 and 2 and repeated every 3 weeks

Bleomycin 30 U IV, days 2, 9, 16, given sequentially with the *cis*-platinum (6 hours after vinblastine), then weekly for a total of 12 doses

Cis-platinum repeated every 21 days for 3–4 courses

Vinblastine is given days 1 and 2 for four courses.

Bleomycin is stopped at a total dose of 360 U (4 courses)

Continuous hydration with normal saline at a rate of at least 100 ml/hr beginning 12 hours prior to first dose is mandatory during 5 days of *cis*-platinum regardless of oral intake.

Drug Administration Schedule for Days 1 and 2

Day 1	Hour 1	Vinblastine
	Hour 6	*Cis*-platinum
Day 2	Hour 1	Vinblastine
	Hour 6	Bleomycin, followed by *cis*-platinum

Indications: Malignant germ cell tumors
Gestational trophoblastic neoplasia (GTN)

Side Effects: Bone marrow depression—especially leukopenia 7–14 days after vinblastine
Renal toxicity, including acute renal failure
Decrease in serum magnesium, calcium, potassium
Moderate to severe nausea and vomiting
High-frequency hearing impairment
Neuropathies
Fever/chills after bleomycin
Alopecia
Cutaneous changes (thickening of nail beds, edema, erythema, hyperpigmentation).
Anorexia—weight loss
Shocklike syndrome
Hypotension
Pulmonary edema
Anaphylaxis
Pulmonary toxicity—pneumonia to fibrosis
Malaise
Paresthesias, myalgias
Phlebitis
Tissue inflammation, necrosis if vinblastine extravasates
Stomatitis

Comments on
Management: Hydrate with normal saline at no less than 100 ml/hr beginning 12 hours before the first dose of *cis*-platinum and continuing throughout 5 days to ensure urinary output of approximately 100 ml/hr. Supplement other electrolytes as needed.
Diuresis with furosemide (Lasix) may be necessary.
Check hemogram.
Check serum electrolytes, creatinine, magnesium, and calcium.
Administer antiemetics.
Administer drugs in free-flowing IV (vinblastine is a vesicant).
Encourage small frequent feedings for anorexia.
Observe bowel and bladder function.

During initial dose of bleomycin, observe vital signs every 15 minutes.

The total dose of bleomycin is not to exceed 360 U.

Obtain pulmonary function tests.

Do not use bleomycin if the carbon monoxide diffusing capacity (DL_{CO}) is less than 50% of predicted or if it drops more than 20% from baseline.

Protocols for Endometrial Sarcoma

Adriamycin 60 mg/m^2 IV every 3 weeks

OR

Cytoxan 1,000 mg/m^2 IV

Vincristine 2 mg IV

Dacarbazine 500 mg/m^2 IV given every 4 weeks

Indications: Uterine sarcomas

Side Effects: Bone marrow depression
Gastrointestinal toxicity
Cardiac toxicity
Liver toxicity
Tissue necrosis
Hemorrhagic cystitis
Alopecia
Neurotoxicity

Comments on
Management: Check hemogram and platelets.
Check liver enzymes.
Double-check vincristine dose if there is a decrease in reflexes or for paresthesias.
Hydrate before and after Cytoxan.
Check ECG.
Consider baseline and serial left ventricular ejection fraction if Adriamycin is used.
Total dose of Adriamycin NOT TO EXCEED 550 mg/m^2.
Administer in a free-flowing IV line.
Encourage frequent voidings.
Administer antiemetics as needed.

Protocol for Rare Sarcomas

Courses 1 and 2 (VADRIC 90)

Vincristine 2 mg/m^2 IV, day 1

Adriamycin 30 mg/m^2 IV, days 1–3

Cytoxan 10 mg/kg, days 1 and 2

Course 3 (VAC)

Vincristine 2 mg/m^2 IV, days 1 and 5

Actinomycin 0.015 mg/kg IV, days 1–5

Cytoxan 10 mg/kg IV, days 1–3

Course 4 (VADRIC 60)

Vincristine 2 mg/m^2 IV, day 1

Adriamycin 30 mg/m^2 IV, days 1 and 2

Cytoxan 10 mg/kg, days 1–3

Give courses 1 and 2 as close together as WBC count recovery will permit (at 4 weeks if possible). Then alternate VAC and VADRIC 60 courses, giving one course every 6 weeks, for a total of 2 years.

NOTE: Maximum dose of vincristine = 2 mg/day
Maximum dose of actinomycin = 0.5 mg/day
Maximum total lifetime dose of Adriamycin 550 mg/m^2 (less if heart irradiated)

Indications: Rare sarcomas (e.g., rhabdomyosarcoma)

Side Effects: Bone marrow depression
Gastrointestinal toxicity
Cardiac toxicity
Liver toxicity
Neurotoxicity
Tissue necrosis
Hemorrhagic cystitis
Alopecia
Dermatitis

Comments on
Management: Check hemogram and platelets.
Check liver enzymes.
Double-check vincristine dose if there is a decrease in reflexes or paresthesias.
Hydrate before and after Cytoxan.

Check ECG.

Consider baseline and serial left ventricular ejection fraction if there are cardiac risk factors.

The total dose of Adriamycin is not to exceed 550 mg/m^2.

Administer in free-flowing IV line.

Encourage frequent voidings.

Administer antiemetics as needed.

Provide oral hygiene.

Protocol for Advanced and/or Recurrent Squamous Cell Cervical Cancer (MOB)

Day 2	Mitomycin-C	10 mg/m^2 IV
Days 1 and 4	Vincristine (Oncovin)	0.5 mg/m^2 IV
Days 1–4	Bleomycin	30 U over 24 hours by continuous IV infusion

Repeat every 6 weeks.

Side Effects: Bone marrow depression
Nausea and vomiting
Fever/chills after bleomycin
Anaphylaxis
Pulmonary toxicity—pneumonitis to fibrosis
Nail changes
Tissue necrosis
Neurotoxicity
Constipation
Alopecia
Stomatitis
Renal toxicity
Anorexia
Hypotension
Pulmonary edema
Shocklike syndrome

Comments on Management: Check hemogram.
Check serum creatinine.
Obtain creatinine clearance if serum creatinine is abnormal or rising.
Obtain pulmonary function tests to include carbon monoxide-diffusing capacity (DL$_{CO}$).

Administer antiemetics.

Consider a permanent central venous catheter.

Administer drugs in a free-flowing IV line.

Encourage small feedings for anorexia.

Observe intestinal and urinary function.

During the initial dose of bleomycin, observe vital signs every 15 minutes.

The total dose of bleomycin is not to exceed 360 U.

Intraperitoneal *Cis*-Platinum

Cis-platinum, 100 mg/m^2, should be mixed in 2 L of normal saline and warmed to body temperature using a blood warmer.

> *Indication:* Recurrent ovarian carcinoma with microscopic or small volume (tumor nodules measure less than 5 mm) residual intraperitoneal disease

Administration:

1. Twelve hours before *cis*-platinum infusion, the patient will begin receiving a continuous IV infusion of 5% dextrose-0.45 NS with 20 mEq/L KCl and 2 g MgSO$_4$/L via a continuous infusion pump (IVAC or IMED) at a rate of 167 ml/hr (1 L every 6 hours). Patients should be premedicated with antiemetics.

2. Prior to *cis*-platinum infusion, the peritoneal cavity should be drained as completely as possible (if an effusion is present), via the Tenchkoff catheter. (If a Port-a-Cath is present, be sure to use a Huber point needle.)

3. *Cis*-platinum infusion: Following 12-hour prehydration, the 2 L of drug-containing fluid should be instilled into the peritoneal cavity as rapidly as possible via the catheter. (Instillation may require 5–30 minutes; if the flow rate is slow, a blood pressure cuff should be placed on the bag containing the drug and inflated to 100 mmHg to speed the flow.)

4. Concurrent with the start of *cis*-platinum infusion, the patient is given an IV bolus infusion (over 10 minutes) of 4 g/m^2 sodium thiosulfate in 250 ml of sterile water, followed by a continuous infusion of 12 g/m^2 mixed in 1 L sterile water over 6 hours.

5. After 4 hours, the peritoneal cavity should again be drained as completely as possible. The catheter should then be flushed with heparinized saline (100 U/ml). Drainage is not mandatory (no adverse con-

sequences other than patient discomfort have been identified even if the full 2 L must be left in the abdomen).

6. From 6–12 hours after intraperitoneal instillation, the patient should continue to receive hydration in the form of 1 L 5% dextrose-0.45 NS with 20 mEq/L KCl and 2 g MgSO$_4$/L. Subsequent hydration is not required but may be advisable depending on the patient's oral intake.

7. Treatment is repeated every 4 weeks or as soon thereafter as the patient has recovered from toxicity.

Side Effects: Abdominal discomfort
Peritonitis
Nephrotoxicity
Ototoxicity
Neuropathies

Comments on
Management: Follow the above protocol.
Check hemogram and platelets.
Check serum creatinine, obtain creatinine clearance if serum creatinine is abnormal or rising.
Check serum electrolyte to include magnesium and calcium.

Protocols for GTN

Nonmetastatic and Low-Risk Gestational Trophoblastic Neoplasia

Primary Regimen

Actinomycin D 0.01 mg/kg/day IV for 5 days (maximum single dose: 0.5 mg)

OR

Methotrexate 0.4 mg/kg/day IM or IV for 5 days (maximum single dose: 30 mg)

Repeat every 3 weeks if granulocytes over 1,500, platelets over 100,000, stomatitis and GI toxicity recovered, and normal aspartate aminotransferase (AST), alanine aminotransferase (ALT), BUN, and serum creatinine.

Continue chemotherapy until:
1. One course past a normal serum β-hCG level
2. hCG levels plateau or begin to rise

Indications: Tissue diagnosis of choriocarcinoma or invasive mole
hCG titers plateauing or rising
Presence of metastasis (other than to liver or brain)
Elevation of hCG level after normal reading

Side Effects: Actinomycin
Nausea, vomiting, diarrhea
Phlebitis, tissue necrosis
Anorexia
Oral and GI ulcerations
Alopecia (minimal)
Bone marrow depression, 1–7 days after dose
Methotrexate
Nausea, vomiting, diarrhea
Oral and GI ulcerations
Hepatic and renal toxicity

Comments on
Management: Administer actinomycin in free-flowing IV.
Monitor intake and output.
Provide oral hygiene.
Check hemogram and platelets.
Check AST (SGOT), ALT (SGPT).
Check serum creatinine and urea nitrogen.
Weekly hCG titers until four normal values are obtained.
Monthly titers for 12 months after normal hCG.
Place on oral contraceptives for 1 year after remission induction.

Alternate Regimens

Actinomycin D 1.25 mg/m^2 IV every 2 weeks

OR

Methotrexate 30 mg/m^2 IM once a week; weekly dose escalated by 5 mg/m^2 at 3-week intervals until a maximum dose of 50 mg/m^2 is achieved

Treatment continues for one course past a normal serum β-hCG titer.

High-Risk GTN
MAC

Methotrexate 0.3 mg/kg IV (max 15 mg)

Actinomycin D 0.01 mg/kg IV (max 0.5 mg)

Cyclophosphamide (Cytoxan) 3–5 mg/kg IV (max 250 mg)

Administer daily for 5 days and repeat every 2–3 weeks.

Indication: High-risk GTN

Side Effects: Bone marrow depression, potentially severe GI toxicity (nausea, stomatitis, diarrhea)
Alopecia
Hemorrhagic cystitis (secondary to Cytoxan metabolites)
Phlebitis, local ulceration (secondary to actinomycin D)

Comments on
Management: Monitor intake and output.
Administer actinomycin in free-flowing IV—STOP if infiltration occurs.
Provide oral hygiene.
Check hemogram and platelets.
Hydrate to prevent hemorrhagic cystitis that can be caused by Cytoxan.
Encourage frequent voidings.

BEP

Day 1	1900 hours *cis*-platinum 50 mg/m^2 IV
Days 1–4	Bleomycin 15 U/24 hr (continuous infusion)
Days 1–4	VP-16 (etoposide) 100 mg/m^2 IV Repeat every 21 days.

Indication: High-risk GTN

Side Effects: Bone marrow depression
Gastrointestinal toxicity
Hypotension
Anaphylactic reaction
Alopecia
Peripheral neuropathy
Nephrotoxicity
Ototoxicity
Pneumonitis, pulmonary fibrosis
Fever/chills after bleomycin
Anorexia
Cutaneous changes (thickening of nails, edema, erythema, hyperpigmentation)

Comments on
Management: Administer VP-16 in 500 ml of normal saline over 1 hour.

Do not give VP-16 by rapid IV push.

Check hemogram and platelets.

Check serum creatinine.

Obtain creatinine clearance if serum creatinine is abnormal or rising.

Check serum electrolytes to include magnesium and calcium.

Administer antiemetics.

Encourage small frequent feedings for anorexia.

During initial dose of bleomycin, observe vital signs every 15 minutes.

Obtain pulmonary function tests.

Do not use bleomycin if carbon monoxide-diffusing capacity (DL_{CO}) is less than 50% of predicted or if it drops more than 20% from baseline.

EMA-CO

Course I (repeated every 14 days)

Day 1	Etoposide	100 mg/m^2 IV
	Dactinomycin	0.5 mg IV
	Methotrexate	100 mg/m^2 IV, 12-hour infusion
Day 2	Etoposide	100 mg/m^2 IV
	Dactinomycin	0.5 mg IV
	Folinic Acid	15 mg IM, every 12 hours for four doses

Course II (repeated every 14 days)

Day 8	Vincristine	1.0 mg/m^2 IV
	Cyclophosphamide	600 mg/m^2 IV

Indications: GTN resistant to MAC protocol and very high-risk metastatic GTN

Side Effects: Bone marrow depression
Gastrointestinal toxicity
Hypotension
Anaphylactic reaction
Alopecia

Peripheral neuropathy
Hemorrhagic cystitis
Neurotoxicity
Phlebitis, tissue necrosis

Comments on
Management: Administer actinomycin and vincristine in free-flowing IV line—STOP if infiltration occurs.
Administer etoposide in 500 ml of normal saline over 1 hour.
Check hemogram and platelets.
Check serum creatinine.
Check serum electrolytes.
Administer antiemetics.
Hydrate before and after Cytoxan.
Encourage frequent voidings.
Monitor intake and output.
Provide oral hygiene.

Modified Bagshawe Regimen

Day 1:	Hydroxyurea 500 mg PO at 0600, 1200, 1800, and 2400 hours
Day 2:	Vincristine 1 mg/m^2 IV at 0700 hours Methotrexate 100 mg/m^2 IV push at 1900 hours Methotrexate 200 mg/m^2 IV infusion over 12 hours starting at 1900 hours Actinomycin D 0.2 mg IV at 1900 hours
Day 3:	Actinomycin D 0.2 mg IV at 1900 hours Cytoxan 500 mg/m^2 IV at 1900 hours Folinic acid 14 mg IM at 1900 hours
Day 4:	Folinic acid 14 mg IM at 0100 hours Folinic acid 14 mg IM at 0700 hours Folinic acid 14 mg IM at 1300 hours Folinic acid 14 mg IM at 1900 hours Actinomycin D 0.5 mg IV at 1900 hours
Day 5:	Folinic acid 14 mg IM at 0100 hours Actinomycin D 0.5 mg IV at 1900 hours
Days 6 & 7:	No treatment

Day 8:   Cytoxan 500 mg/m² IV at 1900 hours
                   Adriamycin 30 mg/m² IV at 1900 hours

Drugs must be given at times ordered.

Monitor toxicity daily.

Repeat treatment course as soon as toxicity permits after 10 days without treatment.

Indication: Gestational trophoblastic neoplasia resistant to other chemotherapy regimens.

Side Effects: Bone marrow depression—potentially severe
              Nausea, vomiting, diarrhea, or constipation
              Stomatitis, mucositis
              Macopapular rash, facial erythema
              Dysuria
              Azotemia, renal failure
              Liver dysfunction—damage
              Neuropathies (e.g., paresthesias, decreased deep tendon reflexes, headache, dizziness)
              Alopecia
              Hemorrhagic cystitis
              Cardiotoxicity

Comments on
Management: Check hemogram, serum electrolytes, serum creatinine, and liver enzymes.
            Check ECG.
            Check creatinine clearance.
            Hydrate.
            Administer antiemetics.
            Provide oral hygiene.
            Check stool for hemocult.
            Administer in free-flowing IV line with good blood return.
            Monitor intake and output.

SUGGESTED READINGS

Alberts DS, Kronmal R, Baker LH, et al: Phase II randomized trial of cisplatin chemotherapy regimens in the treatment of recurrent or metastatic squamous cell cancer of the cervix: A Southwest Oncology Group Study. J Clin Oncol 5:1971, 1987

Ashford AR, Donev I, Tiwari RP, et al: Reversible ocular toxicity related to tamoxifen therapy. Cancer 61:33, 1988

Baker LH, Opipari MI, Wilson H, et al: Mitomycin C, vincristine, and bleomycin therapy for advanced cervical cancer. Obstet Gynecol 52:146, 1978

Bennett WM, Pastore L, Houghton DC: Fatal pulmonary bleomycin toxicity in cisplatin-induced renal failure. Cancer Treatm Rep 64:921, 1980

Blachley JD, Hill JB: Renal and electrolyte disturbances associated with cisplatin. Ann Intern Med 95:628, 1981.

Bristow MR, Lopez MB, Mason JW, et al: Efficiency and cost of cardiac monitoring in patients receiving doxorubicin. Cancer 50:32, 1982

Brucker HW, Dinse GE, Davis TE, et al: A randomized comparison of cyclophosphamide, adriamycin and 5-fluorouracil with triethyelene-thiophosphoramide and methotrexate, both as sequential and as fixed rotational treatment in patients with advanced ovarian cancer. Cancer 55:26, 1985

Budd GT, Webster KD, Reimer RR, et al: Treatment of advanced ovarian cancer with cisplatin, adriamycin, and cyclophosphamide: Effect of treatment and incidence of intracranial metastases. J Surg Oncol 24:192, 1983

Carlson JA Jr, Allegra JC, Day TG Jr, et al: Tamoxifen and endometrial carcinoma: Alterations in estrogen and progesterone receptors in untreated patients and combination hormonal therapy in advanced neoplasia. Am J Obstet Gynecol 149:149, 1984

Conte PF, Bruzzone M, Chiara S, et al: A randomized trial comparing cisplatin plus cyclophosphamide versus cisplatin, doxorubicin, and cyclophosphamide in advanced ovarian cancer. J Clin Oncol 4:965, 1986

Cudmore MA, Silva J Jr, Fekety R, et al: *Clotridium difficile* colitis associated with cancer chemotherapy. Arch Intern Med 142:333, 1982

Curry S, Blessing J, DiSaia P, et al: A prospective randomized comparison of methotrexate, actinomycin D, and cyclophosphamide (MAC) versus modified Bagshawe regimen in "poor-prognosis" gestational trophoblastic disease. Gynecol Oncol 26:407, 1987 (abst)

Davila E, Gardner LB: Clinical value of the creatinine clearance before the administration of chemotherapy with cisplatin. Cancer 60:161, 1987

Decker DG, Fleming TR, Malkasian GD Jr, et al: Cyclophosphamide plus cis-platinum in combination: Treatment program for stage III or IV ovarian carcinoma. Obstet Gynecol 60:481, 1982

Druck MN, Gulenchyn KY, Evans WK, et al: Radionuclide angiography and endomyocardial biopsy in the assessment of doxorubicin cardiotoxicity. Cancer 53:1667, 1984

Einhorn N, Eklund G, Franzen S, et al: Late side effects of chemotherapy in ovarian carcinoma: A cytogenetic, hematologic, and statistical study. Cancer 49:2234, 1982

El Saghir NS, Hawkins KA: Hepatotoxicity following vincristine therapy. Cancer 54:2006, 1984

George M, Pejoric MH, Kramar A, et al: Uterine sarcomas: Prognostic factors and treatment modalities—study on 209 patients. Gynecol Oncol 24:58, 1986

Gershenson DM, Copeland LJ, Kavanagh JJ, et al: Treatment of malignant nondysgerminomatous germ cell tumors of the ovary with vincristine, dactinomycin, and cyclophosphamide. Cancer 56:2756, 1985

Gershenson DM, Copeland LJ, Kavanagh JJ, et al: Treatment of metastatic stromal tumors of the ovary with cisplatin, doxorubicin, and cyclophosphamide. Obstet Gynecol 70:765, 1987

Gershenson DM, Del Junco G, Herson J, et al: Endodermal sinus tumor of the ovary: The M.D. Anderson experience. Obstet Gynecol 61:194, 1983

Gershenson DM, Del Junco G, Silva EG, et al: Immature teratoma of the ovary. Obstet Gynecol 68:624, 1986

Gershenson DM, Kavanagh JJ, Copeland LJ, et al: Treatment of malignant nondysgerminomatous germ cell tumors of the ovary with vinblastine, bleomycin, and cisplatin. Cancer 57:1731, 1986

Gershenson DM, Wharton T, Kline RC, et al: Chemotherapeutic complete remission in patients with metastatic ovarian dysgerminoma: Potential for cure and preservation of reproductive capacity. Cancer 58:2594, 1986

Gonzalez C, Villasanta U: Life-threatening hypocalcemia and hypomagnesemia associated with cisplatin chemotherapy. Obstet Gynecol 59:732, 1982

Gordon AN, Kavanagh JJ, Gershenson DM, et al: Cisplatin, vinblastine, and bleomycin combination therapy in resistant gestational trophoblastic disease. Cancer 58:1407, 1986

Gottlieb JA, Benjamin RS, Baker LH, et al: Role of DTIC (NSC-45388) in the chemotherapy of sarcomas. Cancer Treatm Rep 60:199, 1976

Grosh WM, Jones HW III, Burnett LS, et al: Malignant mixed mesodermal tumors of the uterus and ovary treated with cisplatin-based combination chemotherapy. Gynecol Oncol 25:334, 1986

Hernandez E, Rosenshein NB, Villar J, et al: Alternating multiagent chemotherapy for advanced ovarian cancer. J Surg Oncol 22:87, 1983

Hoffman MS, Roberts WS, Bryson SCP, et al: Treatment of recurrent and metastatic cervical cancer with cis-platin, doxorubicin, and cyclophosphamide. Gynecol Oncol 29:32, 1988

Homesley MD, Blessing JA, Rettenmaier M, et al: Weekly intramuscular methotrexate for nonmetastatic gestational trophoblastic disease. Obstet Gynecol 72:413, 1988

Howell SB, Pfeifle CL, Wung WE, et al: Intraperitoneal cisplatin with systemic thiosulfate protection. Ann Intern Med 97:845, 1982

Howell SB, Zimm S, Markman M, et al: Long-term survival of advanced refractory ovarian carcinoma patients with small-volume disease treated with intraperitoneal chemotherapy. J Clin Oncol 5:1607, 1987

Lovecchio JL, Averette HE, Linchtinger M, et al: Treatment of advanced or recurrent endometrial adenocarcinoma with cyclophosphamide, doxorubicin, cis-platinum, and megestrol acetate. Obstet Gynecol 63:557, 1984

Lucas WE, Markman M, Howell SB: Intraperitoneal chemotherapy for advanced ovarian cancer. Am J Obstet Gynecol 152:474, 1985

Malviya V, Deppe G, Malone J, Jr: Cis-platinum based combination chemotherapy in advanced metastatic mixed mesodermal sarcoma of the uterus. Proc American Society of Clinical Oncology 7:142, 1988 (abst)

McDonald TW, Ruffolo EH: Modern management of gestational trophoblastic disease. Obstet Gynecol Surv 38:67, 1983

Muggia FM, Chia G, Reed LJ, et al: Doxorubicin-cyclophosphamide: Effective chemotherapy for advanced endometrial adenocarcinoma. Am J Obstet Gynecol 128:314, 1977

Muss HB, Jobson VW, Homesley HD, et al: Neoadjuvant therapy for advanced squamous cell carcinoma of the cervix: Cisplatin followed by radiation therapy—a pilot study of the Gynecologic Oncology Group. Gynecol Oncol 26:35, 1987

Newlands ES, Rustin GJS, Gagshawe KD, et al: Weekly EMA/CO chemotherapy for high-risk gestational trophoblastic tumors. Proc American Society of Clinical Oncology 5:112, 1986 (abst)

Omura GA, Major FJ, Blessing JA, et al: A randomized study of Adriamycin with and without dimethyl triazenoimidazole carboxamide in advanced uterine sarcomas. Cancer 52:626, 1983

Ozols RF, Cordeu BJ, Jacob J, et al: High-dose cisplatin in hypertonic saline. Ann Intern Med 100:19, 1984

Ozols RF, Ostchega Y, Myers CE, et al: High-dose cisplatin in hypertonic saline in refractory ovarian cancer. J Clin Oncol 3:1246, 1985

Podratz KC, O'Brien PC, Malkasian GD Jr, et al: Effects of progestational agents in treatment of endometrial carcinoma. Obstet Gynecol 66:106, 1985

Ritch PS, Louie AC: Skin rash following therapy with Mitomycin C. Cancer 54:32, 1984

Rotmensch J, Rosenshein N, Donehower R, et al: Plasma methotrexate levels in patients with gestational trophoblastic neoplasia treated by two methotrexate regimens. Am J Obstet Gynecol 148:730, 1984

Rudolph R, Larson DL: Etiology and treatment of chemotherapeutic agent extravasation injuries: A review. J Clin Oncol 5:1116, 1987

Schlaerth JB, Morrow CP, Nalick RH, et al: Single-dose Actinomycin D in the treatment of postmolar trophoblastic disease. Gynecol Oncol 19:53, 1984

Schwartz P: Combination chemotherapy in the management of ovarian germ cell malignancies. Obstet Gynecol 64:564, 1984

Shuman RD, Ettinger DS, Abeloff MD, et al: Comparative analysis of noninvasive cardiac parameters in the detection and evaluation of adriamycin cardiotoxicity. Johns Hopkins Med J 149:57, 1981

Slayton RE, Park RC, Silverberg SG, et al: Vincristine, dactinomycin, and cyclophosphamide in the treatment of malignant germ cell tumors of the ovary: A Gynecologic Oncology Group study. A final report. Cancer 56:243, 1985

Sorbe B: Radiotherapy and/or chemotherapy as adjuvant treatment of uterine sarcomas. Gynecol Oncol 20:281, 1985

Surwit EA, Alberts DS, Christian CD, et al: Poor-prognosis gestational trophoblastic disease: An update. Obstet Gynecol 64:21, 1984

Taylor MH, DePetrillo AD, Turner AR: Vinblastine, bleomycin, and cisplatin in malignant germ cell tumors of the ovary. Cancer 56:1341, 1985

Thompson SW, Davis LE, Kornfeld M, et al: Cisplatin neuropathy: Clinical, electrophysiologic, morphologic, and toxicologic studies. Cancer 54:1269, 1984

Trope C, Johnsson J-E, Simonsen E, et al: Treatment of recurrent endometrial adenocarcinoma with a combination of doxorubicin and cisplatin. Am J Obstet Gynecol 149:379, 1984

Quinn MA, Campbell JJ: Tamoxifen therapy in advanced/recurrent endometrial carcinoma. Gynecol Oncol 32:1, 1989

Valavaara R, Nordman E: Renal complications of mitomycin C therapy with special reference to the total dose. Cancer 55:47, 1985

Verweij J, Van Zanten T, Souren T, et al: Prospective study on the dose relationship of mitomycin C-induced interstitial pneumonitis. Cancer 60:756, 1987

Von Hoff DD, Layard MW, Basa P, et al: Risk factors for doxorubicin-induced congestive heart failure. Ann Intern Med 91:710, 1979

Walther PJ, Rossitch E Jr, Bullard DE: The development of Lhermitte's sign during cisplatin chemotherapy: Possible drug-induced toxicity causing spinal cord demyelation. Cancer 60:2170, 1987

Weed JC Jr, Barnard DE, Currie JL, et al: Chemotherapy with the modified Bagshawe protocol for poor prognosis metastatic trophoblastic disease. Obstet Gynecol 59:377, 1982

Weiss RB, Bruno S: Hypersensitivity reactions to cancer chemotherapeutic agents. Ann Intern Med 94:66, 1981

Williams SD, Birch R, Einhorn LH, et al: Treatment of disseminated germ-cell tumors with cisplatin, bleomycin, and either vinblastine or etoposide. N Engl J Med 316:1435, 1987

8

Perioperative Care of the Patient Undergoing Radical Hysterectomy

The radical abdominal hysterectomy, bilateral pelvic lymphadenectomy, is an operation designed to treat those patients who have limited invasive carcinoma of the cervix, classified as stage IA with lymphovascular invasion, stage IB, or early stage IIA, or for selected patients with stage II endometrial cancer. This operation involves extensive dissection (Fig. 8-1). Meticulous perioperative care results in reduced morbidity. What follows are our standards for the perioperative care of these patients.

VITAL SIGNS

PREOPERATIVE
Temperature, pulse, respirations, and blood pressure are taken before the patient is transported to the operating room. These readings are recorded on a flowchart.

POSTOPERATIVE
Temperature, pulse, respirations, and blood pressure are taken every 4 hours for the first 48 hours postoperatively and are recorded on the flowchart. Thereafter, temperature, pulse, and respirations are taken three times a day (e.g., 0800, 1600, 2400 hours), with blood pressure taken daily unless the patient's condition warrants more frequent monitoring.

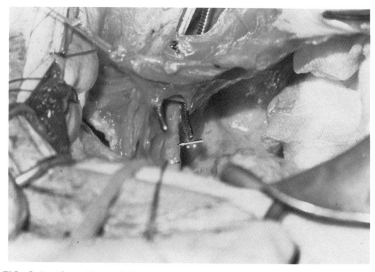

FIG. 8-1. Dissection of the ureter (arrow) during a radical abdominal hysterectomy.

INTAKE AND OUTPUT

PREOPERATIVE

A flowchart is started the evening before the day of surgery and is sent to the operating room with the patient. The IV infusion that is begun preoperatively as well as all output is recorded on this chart.

POSTOPERATIVE

Intake and output are recorded with 4-hour summaries until the discontinuation of all IV fluids and catheters, unless otherwise ordered.

PHYSICAL PARAMETERS

PREOPERATIVE

The patient's weight is obtained and recorded on the flowchart before she is sent to the operating room.

POSTOPERATIVE

Weight is obtained every day and recorded on the flowchart. Abdominal girth and calf measurements are obtained daily and recorded on the flow chart until the fifth postoperative day.

RESPIRATORY CARE

PREOPERATIVE

Incentive spirometry is taught preoperatively to all patients. The patient is also given instructions in turning, coughing, and deep breathing.

POSTOPERATIVE

Incentive spirometry is done every 4 hours for 72 hours postoperatively or until the patient is fully ambulatory. Turning, coughing, and deep breathing with nursing supervision is done every 4 hours.

AMBULATION

PREOPERATIVE

The patient will be informed and will be instructed on the importance of progressive ambulation during the postoperative period.

POSTOPERATIVE

The patient is out of bed the night of surgery. Beginning on the first postoperative day, the patient is ambulated at least three times a day.

INDWELLING CATHETER CARE

PREOPERATIVE

Instruction is given to the patient concerning the fact that she will have a transurethral or a suprapubic catheter in place for a minimum of 14 days.

POSTOPERATIVE

The patient with a Foley catheter is given standard catheter care: periurethral hygiene followed by cleansing of the catheter with Betadine solution from the external urethral meatus to the junction of the Foley catheter with the drainage system. In the patient with a suprapubic catheter, the incisional area and the catheter are cleansed with Betadine from the skin margin to the junction with the draining system.

The transurethral catheter is removed on day 14. The patient has residual urines checked after the first and third voidings. If the residual urine is less that 50 ml, no further catheterization is required. If the residual urine is greater than 100 ml after the third voiding, the Foley catheter is reinserted for a period of 2 days before another attempt at removal and obtaining residual urine measurements is made.

If a suprapubic catheter is used, the catheter is clamped after 14 days. The patient is instructed to void, and on the first and third voidings the residual amount of urine is measured. If these are greater than 100 ml, the catheter is left unclamped for a period of 48 hours before the residual urine is again measured.

Upon removal of the catheter, terminal urine is obtained for culture and sensitivity and urinalysis. We obtain an excretory urogram approximately 4 weeks after surgery.

THROMBOEMBOLISM PROPHYLAXIS

PREOPERATIVE

The patient receives 5,000 U of heparin subcutaneously (SC) 4 hours prior to the scheduled surgery. Alternatively, a sequential pneumatic calf-compressor device is used during the surgery.

POSTOPERATIVE

The patient receives 5,000 U of heparin SC every 12 hours, until fully ambulatory. This commences 4 hours after completion of surgery. Patients should be monitored for heparin-induced idiopathic thrombocytopenia. Alternatively, a sequential pneumatic calf-compressor device is used postoperatively until the patient is fully ambulatory.

WOUND CARE

PREOPERATIVE

Instruction is given to the patient concerning the fact that she will have an abdominal incision and a large pressure dressing that will be removed on the first or second postoperative day. A vaginal Betadine douche is given the evening before surgery. The patient is asked to shower with Hibiclens the evening before surgery. If abdominal or pubic hair will interfere with the surgery, clipping or shaving is done in the operating room. Clipping is preferred.

POSTOPERATIVE

The incisional pressure dressing is removed on the first or second postoperative day. The incision is inspected for any signs of separation or inflammation and is cleansed thoroughly with hydrogen peroxide and saline to remove all residual iodine, blood, and adhesive material. A Telfa bandage is placed over the incision for an additional 24 hours, after which the incision is left uncovered.

INTRAVENOUS FLUIDS

An IV line is started with a short Silastic catheter (e.g., Angiocath) the day before surgery or early on the day of surgery. The patient is informed that an IV infusion will be maintained until she is able to tolerate her diet. If not allergic, 200 mg of doxycycline (Vibramycin) is given IV on call to the operating room.

DRAINS

PREOPERATIVE

The patient is informed that closed suction drains are to be left in the pelvis and brought out through separate stab incisions in the flanks.

POSTOPERATIVE

The output from each individual drain is monitored. The drains are left in for a minimum of 48–72 hours and until the drainage from each drain is less than 50 ml in 24 hours.

INTESTINAL PREPARATION

The physician discusses with the patient the purpose and importance of the intestinal preparation. The GoLYTELY intestinal preparation described in Appendix I is initiated. (Substitutions may be made by the physician.)

CARDIORESPIRATORY MONITORING

Arterial blood gases (ABGs) are obtained before surgery. Pulmonary function tests are obtained if indicated. An electrocardiogram and chest radiograph are ordered for the first postoperative day. A hemogram and serum electrolytes are obtained on postoperative days 1 and 3 and as indicated. Two to 4 units of packed red blood cells (PRBC) should be available.

SUGGESTED READINGS

Allen HH, Nisker JA, Anderson RJ: Primary surgical treatment in one hundred ninety-five cases of stage IB carcinoma of the cervix. Am J Obstet Gynecol 143:581, 1982

Clarke-Pearson DL, Synan IS, Hinshaw WM, et al: Prevention of postoperative venous thromboembolism by external pneumatic calf compression in patients with gynecologic malignancy. Obstet Gynecol 631:92, 1984

DiSaia PJ: The case against the surgical concept of *en bloc* dissection for certain malignancies of the reproductive tract. Cancer 60:2025, 1987

Farquharson DI, Orr JW Jr: Prophylaxis against thromboembolism in gynecologic patients. J Reprod Med 29:845, 1984

Garner JS, Emori TG, Haley RW: Operating room practices for the control of infection in U.S. hospitals, October 1976 to July 1977. Surg Gynecol Obstet 155:873, 1982

Miyazawa K, Hernandez E, Dillon MB: Prophylactic topical cefamandole in radical hysterectomy. Int J Gynecol Obstet 25:133, 1987

Rosenshein NB, Ruth JC, Villar J, et al: A prospective randomized study of doxycycline as a prophylactic antibiotic in patients undergoing radical hysterectomy. Gynecol Oncol 15:201, 1983

Wallin TE, Malkasian GF Jr, Gaffey TA, et al: Stage II cancer of the endometrium: A pathologic and clinical study. Gynecol Oncol 18:1, 1984

9

Perioperative Care of the Patient Undergoing Radical Vulvectomy

The radical vulvectomy, bilateral inguinal lymphadenectomy, is used for the treatment of invasive carcinoma of the vulva. This operation includes en bloc dissection of the inguinal-femoral groin nodes with their connecting lymphatic channels, together with the vulva (labia minora, labia majora, clitoris, perineal body) (Fig. 9-1). The vulvar incision is carried down to the inferior fascia of the urogenital diaphragm. In an effort to reduce morbidity while maintaining the same cure rates, less extensive procedures are being performed in selected cases (Fig. 9-2). Meticulous perioperative care further reduces operative morbidity and mortality. What follows are suggested standards of care for the perioperative management of these patients.

VITAL SIGNS

PREOPERATIVE

Temperature, pulse, respirations, and blood pressure are taken before the patient is transported to the operating room. These readings are recorded on a flowchart.

POSTOPERATIVE

Temperature, pulse, respirations, and blood pressure are taken every 4 hours for 48 hours and are recorded on the flowchart. After the initial 48 hours, the temperature, pulse, and respirations are taken three times a day (e.g., 0800, 1600, and 2400 hours), with

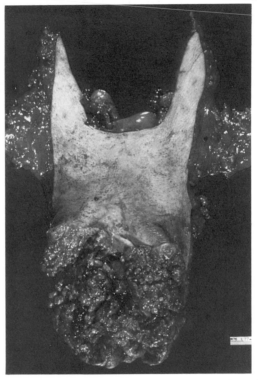

FIG. 9-1. Radical vulvectomy specimen. En bloc dissection of superficial and deep inguinal nodes with the overlying skin, mons, and vulva.

blood pressure taken daily unless the patient's condition requires more frequent monitoring.

INTAKE AND OUTPUT

PREOPERATIVE

All intake and output is measured and recorded on the flow-chart, beginning with initiation of the infusion.

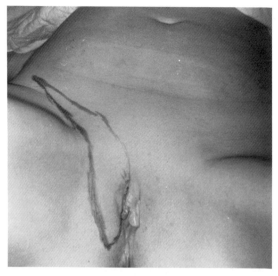

FIG. 9-2. Outline of incision to be made on patient with stage I squamous cell carcinoma of the right labium majus.

POSTOPERATIVE

Intake and output are recorded with 4-hour summaries until all IV fluids, catheters and drains are discontinued. The output from each drain is measured and recorded separately.

PHYSICAL PARAMETERS

PREOPERATIVE

The patient's weight and abdominal, thigh, and calf girths are obtained preoperatively and recorded on the flowchart.

POSTOPERATIVE

Weight and abdominal, thigh, and calf girths are obtained daily and recorded on the flowchart until the sixth postoperative day.

RESPIRATORY CARE

PREOPERATIVE

All patients are taught incentive spirometry, as well as turning, coughing, and deep breathing prior to surgery.

POSTOPERATIVE

Incentive spirometry is done every 2 hours while the patient is awake until the patient is ambulatory. Positioning, coughing, and deep breathing with nursing supervision is done every 4 hours.

AMBULATION

PREOPERATIVE

The patient is instructed in

1. How to perform isometric leg exercises
2. The use of a footboard
3. The importance of these exercises
4. The reason for, and importance of, bed rest during the immediate post-operative period (reduce tension on the incision),
5. The importance of slow but progressive ambulation beginning 3–4 days postoperatively

POSTOPERATIVE

The patient remains in bed for 2–3 days postoperatively. Leg exercises (isometric and using a footboard) are done at least every 4 hours. When the patient is able to be out of bed, progressive ambulation is initiated with nursing supervision, and with the use of a walker. Intermittent pneumatic calf compression is used until the patient is fully ambulatory.

INDWELLING CATHETER CARE

PREOPERATIVE

Instruction is given the patient regarding the fact that she will have a transurethral catheter in place for 3–5 days after surgery, or until she is able to void.

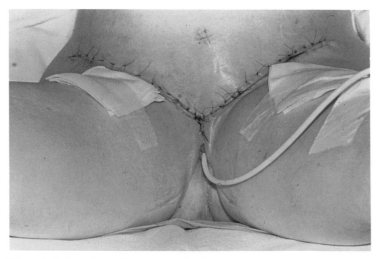

FIG. 9-3. Suture line after a radical vulvectomy.

POSTOPERATIVE

The patient is given standard catheter care: periurethral hygiene followed by cleansing of the catheter with Betadine solution from the external urethral meatus to the junction of the Foley catheter; a terminal urine is sent for culture and sensitivity and urinalysis. The patient's voiding pattern is monitored (frequency and amount; determine continency and ability to void).

THROMBOEMBOLISM PROPHYLAXIS
PREOPERATIVE

The patient receives 5,000 U of heparin subcutaneously (SC) 4 hours prior to the scheduled surgery time. Alternatively, a sequential pneumatic calf-compressor device is used.

POSTOPERATIVE

The patient receives 5,000 U of heparin SC every 12 hours beginning 4 hours after the completion of the surgery and until she is ambulatory. The heparin injections should not be administered below the umbilicus. Alternatively, a pneumatic calf-compressor device is used postoperatively until fully ambulatory.

WOUND CARE

PREOPERATIVE

The patient is instructed that she will have bilateral groin incisions and a vulvar incision and that the surgical dressing will be removed the morning after the operation (Fig. 9-3). A Betadine douche is given the evening before surgery. The patient is asked to shower using Hibiclens the evening before surgery. Soap sud enemas are given that evening. Clipping or shaving of the surgical site is done in the operating room.

POSTOPERATIVE

The surgical dressing is removed on the first postoperative day. The incisions are inspected for any signs of inflammation or separation and are cleansed thoroughly with hydrogen peroxide and saline to remove all residual iodine, blood, and adhesive material. Antibiotic ointment (e.g., Bacitracin) is applied to the incisions and no dressing is applied. This suture line care is performed by the nursing staff every 8 hours.

INTRAVENOUS FLUIDS

An IV infusion is started early on the day of surgery. The patient is instructed that she will have IV infusion until she is able to tolerate her diet.

DRAINS

PREOPERATIVE

The patient is informed that closed suction drains will be left in the groin incisions but that they will come out through separate stab incisions.

POSTOPERATIVE

The output from each individual drain is monitored. The drains are left in for a minimum of 48–72 hours and until drainage is less than 25 ml per drain in 24 hours.

CARDIORESPIRATORY MONITORING

Arterial blood gases (ABGs) are obtained before surgery. Pulmonary function tests are obtained if indicated. An electrocardiogram and chest radiograph are ordered for the first postoperative day. An intensive care unit bed should be reserved prior to surgery. Two to 4 units of packed red blood cells (PRBC) should be available.

SUGGESTED READINGS

Clarke-Pearson DL, Synan IS, Hinshaw WM, et al: Prevention of postoperative venous thromboembolism by external pneumatic calf compression in patients with gynecologic malignancy. Obstet Gynecol 63:92, 1984

Farquharson DI, Orr JW Jr: Prophylaxis against thromboembolism in gynecologic patients. J Reprod Med 29:845, 1984

Garner JS, Emori TG, Haley RW: Operating room practices for the control of infection in U.S. hospitals, October 1976 to July 1977. Surg Gynecol Obstet 155:873, 1982

Hacker NF, Berek JS, Lagasse LD, et al: Individualization of treatment for stage I squamous cell vulvar carcinoma. Obstet Gynecol 63:155, 1984

10

Perioperative Care of the Patient Undergoing Intracavitary Irradiation

Patients are treated with intracavitary (Fig. 10-1) and occasionally interstitial radiation therapy for invasive cancer of the female genital tract, either as primary treatment or as adjuvant therapy. The medical personnel taking care of these patients should be knowledgeable in the basic principles of radiation biology, radiation physics, and radiation safety. A discussion of these principles is beyond the scope of this manual. What follows are standards of care for the patient receiving brachytherapy. They are intended to decrease patient morbitity and maintain medical personnel radiation exposure to a minimum.

PREOPERATIVE PREPARATION

The patient is given a cleansing enema and Betadine douche the evening before the application of intracavitary radiation. The patient is given 2 g of a first-generation cephalosporin (e.g., Ancef), on call to the operating room, except to patients with an allergy to penicillin. The cephalosporin is continued at 1 g every 6 hours until removal of the implant.

VITAL SIGNS

PREOPERATIVE

Temperature, pulse, respirations, and blood pressure are obtained and recorded before the patient goes to surgery for placement of the intracavitary implant.

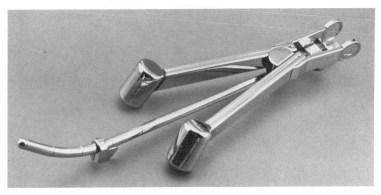

FIG. 10-1. Fletcher-Suit afterloading applicator (tandem and ovoids) used for intracavitary irradiation of gynecologic malignancies.

POSTOPERATIVE

Temperature, pulse, and respirations are taken three times a day (e.g., 0800, 1600, and 2400 hours).

INTAKE AND OUTPUT

PREOPERATIVE

The patient should have nothing by mouth (NPO) for 8 hours prior to the procedure. A flowchart is started before the patient is sent to the operating room. The IV fluid that is given preoperatively is recorded on this chart.

POSTOPERATIVE

The patient is placed on a low-residue diet when she is fully awake. In order to keep radiation exposure to a minimum, IV fluids are administered through a mechanical infusion pump (e.g., IMED, IVAC), and the volume infused is recorded every 8 hours. Intake and output are recorded on the flowchart.

THROMBOEMBOLISM PROPHYLAXIS

PREOPERATIVE

The patient receives 5,000 U of subcutaneous (SC) heparin every 12 hours in the upper extremities while the radiation source is in place. Consider the use of a pneumatic calf-compressor device.

AMBULATION

PREOPERATIVE

The patient is informed that after the placement of the applicators and sources, she will be on bed rest and that her mobility in bed will be limited as described below.

POSTOPERATIVE

The patient must lie flat in her bed at all time. The head of the bed may be elevated 30 degrees during meals. Legs may be moved freely, but it is imperative that the hips remain flat on the bed. If the patient has a mold or cylinder that is sutured in place, more liberal movement may be allowed with the written approval of a gynecologic oncologist or a radiation oncologist. Under no circumstance are patients permitted to sit up or get out of bed with the applicators and sources in place without the written permission of a gynecologic oncologist or radiation oncologist.

RESPIRATORY CARE

Because of the very short duration of the anesthesia and the risks of radiation exposure, no specific respiratory protocol is required after the patient has recovered from anesthesia.

INTRAVENOUS FLUIDS

PREOPERATIVE

Intravenous fluids are initiated the morning of the application.

POSTOPERATIVE

Intravenous fluids to keep the vein open are continued for as long as the patient has the intracavitary radiation in place. This can be substituted for a heparin lock if the patient is tolerating her meals. Ancef (or similar cephalosporin), 1 g, is given IV every 6 hours until the removal of the radiation sources and applicators.

URETHRAL CATHETERIZATION

PREOPERATIVE

The patient is informed that a Foley catheter will be inserted and will remain in place until the removal of the intracavitary radiation.

POSTOPERATIVE

The patient has a Foley inserted at the time of the insertion of the instruments. The catheter remains in place until the radiation sources and applicators are removed. When the catheter is removed, a terminal urine is sent for culture and sensitivity and urinalysis. Standard catheter care with Betadine is not done because of the risk of radiation exposure.

COMFORT MEASURES

In order to ensure the patient's comfort and prevent complications, several measures should be considered:

1. Use of fleece blankets

2. Use of an airflow mattress (e.g., Lapidus, Gaymar) for the extremely thin patient or for the patient with skin changes from external beam therapy
3. Liberal use of pain medication and sedatives as needed
4. Changing the bed linen, but only when wet or soiled

INSERTION OF THE SOURCES

FLETCHER APPLICATORS (AFTERLOADING)

The sources are inserted after the patient has returned to a room approved by the radiation safety officer.

VAGINAL MOLD

The sources are inserted in the operating room when the mold is sutured in place.

INTERSTITIAL IRIDIUM

Sources are placed in the radiation therapy department before the patient returns to the ward.

PATIENT ROOMS

The rooms are marked with radiation warning signs. No linen or gowns are to be removed from the room until the room has been cleared by the radiation safety officer and an order written that the removal of material is safe.

VISITORS

No visitors are permitted during the time that the patient has the radiation sources in place. Exceptions need to be approved by the gynecologic oncologist or radiation oncologist. No allied medical personnel (phlebotomists, technicians, housekeepers, dietary personnel) are permitted in the room while the patient has active sources.

RADIOACTIVE SOURCES

To ensure that the radiation sources are in place, the applicator is checked in the morning, midday, and evening.

RADIATION SAFETY INCIDENTS

Radiation safety incidents include any of the following:

1. Change in patient's position without written consent of a gynecologic oncologist or radiation oncologist
2. Displacement of applicator and/or source
3. Discovery of source out of applicator or part of applicator loose in bed
4. Removal of catheter by patient
5. Temperature elevation over 100.4°F (38°C)
6. Presence of abdominal pain/peritoneal signs
7. Patient develops marked confusion or agitation

Any incident that occurs while the patient has the sources and applicators in place is reported IMMEDIATELY to the gynecologic oncologist, or radiation oncologist.

POST-TREATMENT MANAGEMENT

After the radiation sources are removed, the catheter is removed. The patient is given a Betadine douche, and 2 g of estrogen-based vaginal cream (e.g., Premarin) (if not an adenocarcinoma) is given intravaginally. The IV infusion, antibiotics, and heparin are discontinued.

SUGGESTED READINGS

Clarke-Pearson DL, Synan IS, Hinshaw WM, et al: Prevention of postoperative venous thromboembolism by external pneumatic calf compression in patients with gynecologic malignancy. Obstet Gynecol 63:92, 1984

Farquharson DI, Orr JW Jr: Prophylaxis against thromboembolism in gynecologic patients. J Reprod Med 29:845, 1984

Lichter AS, Dillon MB, Rosenshein NB, et al: The use of custom molds for intracavitary treatment of carcinoma of the cervix. Int J Radiat Oncol biol Phys 4:873, 1978

11

Hickman Catheter Care

INDICATIONS

The basic indication for a long-term venous catheter is prolonged venous access:

1. Long-term parenteral nutrition
2. Prolonged parenteral therapy for malignancies with exhaustion of peripheral veins or frequent chemotherapy that can only be given through a central vein
3. Antibiotic treatment of serious infections when peripheral venous access is exhausted
4. Bone marrow transplantation

Any patient who does not require long-term parenteral nutrition, antibiotics, or chemotherapy but who has exhausted her peripheral venous access should be considered for placement of a temporary central venous line. The risks of a temporary central venous line are less than those of a long-term venous catheter.

HICKMAN AND BROVIAC CATHETER

DESCRIPTION

The Hickman catheter is an indwelling large-diameter (1.6 mm) Silastic right atrial catheter. It provides long-term venous access for delivery of infusions and aspiration of blood samples. The Broviac catheter differs in that its lumen is only 1.0 mm in diameter, making aspiration of blood samples more difficult.

PURPOSE

The purpose of the catheter is to facilitate venous access in those patients whose venous system is compromised due to the disease process as well as in those patients who require long-term therapy, e.g., continuous chemotherapy infusions, total parenteral nutrition (TPN).

CATHETER INSERTION

The catheter is 90 cm in length and has a Dacron cuff located approximately 30 cm from the catheter hub. The insertion of the catheter is done in the operating room under sterile conditions. For the cephalic vein cutdown, an incision is made over the deltopectoral groove in order to locate the cephalic vein. Another approach may be the anterolateral neck to expose the external jugular vein. A subcutaneous tunnel is formed from this incision extending downward to form an exit site midway down the anterior wall of the chest between the nipples. The catheter length is then estimated and trimmed to the correct size. The catheter is threaded through the subcutaneous tunnel and enters the selected vein. The catheter is then threaded further, until the tip is positioned in the junction of the superior vena cava and right atrium. The location of the tip of the catheter is verified by fluoroscopy or portable radiography before the incisions are closed. If the patient's platelet count is less than 50,000, a platelet transfusion may be indicated before or during insertion of the catheter.

ALTERNATE ROUTE

The internal jugular vein is an alternate route for entering the superior vena cava. An incision is made over the sternocleidomastoid muscle in order to locate the vein. The entrance site is sutured closed, and a sterile dressing is applied.

DACRON CUFF

As the healing process occurs, the Dacron cuff (located in the subcutaneous tunnel) will adhere to the tissue. The purpose of the cuff is twofold:

1. It anchors the catheter in position.
2. It may serve as a barrier to external ascending infection.

TOTALLY IMPLANTABLE CATHETERS

A modification to the Hickman catheter is the attachment of an infusion port. This infusion port is implanted subcutaneously, accessed by the use of a Huber needle. Therefore, unlike the Hickman catheter, there is no external tubing. The totally implantable Silastic catheter systems (e.g., Port-A-Cath, Norport) require less care. Flushing with heparinized saline needs to be done only immediately before or after each use or once a month. No dressing is needed. Lower catheter-related infections have been reported with the totally implanted catheters.

Complications unique to the totally implanted system exist. These include erosion of the infusion port through the skin, extravasation due to dislodgement of the Huber needle used to access the port, and catheter embolization due to disconnection of the catheter from the port. This last complication is seen with the Port-A-Cath system. This system has the Silastic catheter secured to the port with a stainless steel slip ring over the catheter. At the time of implantation, malalignment of the slip ring may lead to catheter dislodgement from the port.

The totally implantable systems are 10 times more expensive than the Hickman. Complications common to the Hickman and the totally implantable catheters include infection, thrombosis, catheter migration, and catheter occlusion. Although the guidelines that follow are designed to avoid Hickman catheter-related complications, adherence to those guidelines that also apply to the totally implantable systems will reduce morbidity and increase catheter longevity.

GUIDELINES FOR HICKMAN
CATHETER CARE

GENERAL GUIDELINES

1. All catheters are inserted in the operating room under controlled, sterile conditions.

2. After insertion of the catheter, the nurse is responsible for the following activities associated with the care of the catheter:
   a. Maintaining patency of the catheter by proper flushing and capping technique
   b. Aseptic dressing care
   c. Identification of complications
3. Upon returning from the operating room, if fluids are not already infusing, the nurse will either flush with heparinized saline and cap the catheter or administer a continuous infusion.
4. The heparinized saline solution contains 100 U of heparin per ml; 3 ml is used to flush the catheter.
5. If the catheter is capped with no intermittent infusion, the catheter must be routinely flushed once every other day with heparinized saline.
6. The catheter must be flushed with heparinized saline after administering blood products.
7. The catheter must be flushed with heparinized saline after drawing samples.
8. Should catheter occlusion or damage occur, the nurse should immediately notify the responsible physician.
9. All continuous infusions should be regulated by a mechanical pump (e.g., IMED, IVAC) at a rate of at least 21 ml/hr.
10. All IV tubing connected to the catheter should be changed every 24 hours.
11. All injection caps should be changed every other day.
12. Each time an injection cap is removed, it must be replaced with a new sterile one.
13. Luer lock extension tubing should always be connected to the catheter when running a continuous infusion.
14. Luer lock syringes should not be used to flush the catheter.
15. If the catheter is capped, it must be clamped at all times with a clean cannula clamp.
16. Intermittent infusions such as antibiotics may be given through the injection cap using a 1-inch 22-gauge needle.
17. Scissors should never be used near the catheter.
18. Only a cannula clamp should be used to clamp the catheter, and no other type of clamps (e.g., Kelly).
19. The site where the clamp is applied should be rotated.
20. An additional cannula clamp is always taped to the wall in the patient's room.

CATHETER FLUSHING

General Guidelines

1. If the catheter is not being used for infusates, it must be flushed every other day.
2. The cannula clamp must always be secured on the catheter.
3. The injection cap must always be secured on the catheter and changed every other day.

Equipment

1. Heparinized saline (3 ml) in syringe
2. Alcohol wipes
3. Sterile 1-inch 22-gauge needle
4. New injection cap if necessary

Procedure

1. Wash hands.
2. Explain the procedure to the patient.
3. Prepare the catheter injection cap with an alcohol pad by thoroughly scrubbing and allowing it to dry.
4. Insert the 22-gauge needle of the syringe with heparinized saline into the center of the injection cap.
5. Remove the cannula clamp.
6. With slow steady pressure, inject 3 ml of heparinized saline.
7. While pushing the last 0.5 ml of heparinized solution, simultaneously clamp the catheter with the cannula clamp.
8. Remove the needle from the catheter.
9. Wipe the injection cap with alcohol.

DRAWING BLOOD

General Guidelines

1. All mechanical pumps (e.g., IMED, IVAC) should be turned off before drawing blood.
2. The first 8 ml of blood drawn may be sent for blood cultures if required. No blood needs to be discarded when drawing a blood culture.
3. If blood is to be discarded, draw off 7 ml from adults and 5 ml from children.
4. Always remove injection cap to draw blood.

5. Always clamp catheter before opening the line.

Equipment

1. Ten-ml syringe
2. Necessary syringes for blood drawing
3. Heparinized saline (3 ml) in syringe
4. Sterile gloves
5. Alcohol wipes
6. Normal saline (5 ml) in a syringe
7. Sterile injection cap
8. Cannula clamp
9. Sterile needle with needle cover

Procedure

1. Wash hands.
2. Explain the procedure to the patient.
3. Place the patient in the supine position, raising the bed to a comfortable working position.
4. Assemble equipment on the bedside table.
5. Turn off the mechanical pump (e.g., IMED, IVAC) if one is being used.
6. Put on gloves.
7. Clamp the catheter with cannula clamp.
8. If an infusion was running through the catheter, disconnect the IV line at distal portion of catheter and place a sterile needle with cover on the end of the IV line. If the catheter was capped, remove the cap.
9. Clean the end of the catheter with alcohol.
10. Connect the 10-ml syringe to the catheter.
11. Unclamp the catheter and slowly draw off the necessary amount of blood for discard or culture.
12. Reclamp the catheter and connect the new syringe to draw all necessary blood.
13. After blood has been drawn, clamp the catheter and connect the syringe with 5 ml of normal saline.
14. Flush the catheter slowly with 5 ml of saline.
15. Clamp the catheter with the cannula clamp.
16. Disconnect the saline syringe and connect the syringe containing 3 ml of heparinized saline.
17. Unclamp the catheter.
18. Flush the catheter slowly with the heparinized saline.

19. Clamp the catheter as you are pushing the last 0.5 ml of solution into the catheter.
20. Disconnect the syringe and connect the IV line of continuous infusate back to the catheter or place the sterile cap on top if the catheter is not being used.
21. Remove the cannula clamp from the catheter if an infusion is to be given.
22. Turn on the mechanical pump (e.g., IMED, IVAC).
23. Secure the catheter and IV line junction with adhesive tape.

Note: If blood is being drawn for culture a peripheral culture should be obtained as well.

INTERMITTENT INFUSATES

Equipment
1. IV infusate
2. IV tubing
3. One-inch 22-gauge needles
4. Sterile injection cap if necessary
5. Heparinized saline (3 ml)
6. Alcohol wipes

Procedure
1. Ensure that the catheter is clamped.
2. Wash hands.
3. Remove the cap from the IV fluid container and clean the rubber stopper with alcohol.
4. Aseptically spike the IV fluid bottle and run the solution through the line.
5. Connect the 1-inch 22-gauge needle to IV tubing.
6. Clean the injection cap with alcohol wipe and allow to dry.
7. Insert the needle into the injection cap and secure it with tape.
8. Remove the cannula clamp from the catheter.
9. Infuse the IV solution over the designated time.
10. When the solution was infused, clamp the catheter with a cannula clamp.
11. Disconnect the IV tubing and needle from the injection cap.
12. Wipe the injection cap with alcohol and allow to dry.
13. Routine flushing procedure (see the section *Catheter Flushing*, steps 4–9).
14. Replace the injection cap every 24 hours.

CONTINUOUS INFUSION

Equipment

1. Infusate
2. IV administration tubing
3. Sterile mechanical pump cassette
4. Filter (if necessary)
5. Sterile stopcock
6. Luer lock tubing
7. Mechanical infusion pump

Procedure

Catheter Connected to Continuous Infusions

1. Wash hands.
2. Uncap the IV infusate bottle and wipe the rubber stopper thoroughly with alcohol and allow to dry.
3. Aseptically spike bottle.
4. Connect tubing, cassette, and stopcock.
5. Secure connections with tape.
6. Clamp the catheter with a cannula clamp.
7. Turn off mechanical pump with the solution to be discarded.
8. Purge a new IV solution through the pump.
9. Disconnect IV tubing from the catheter.
10. Wipe the catheter hub with alcohol.
11. Connect new IV tubing to the catheter hub.
12. Release the clamp.
13. Turn on the pump.

Capped Catheter

1. Same as steps 1–5 above.
2. Ensure that the catheter is clamped.
3. Remove the injection cap.
4. Wipe the distal portion of catheter with an alcohol wipe.
5. Connect IV tubing.
6. Secure the connection with tape.
7. Remove the cannula clamp.
8. Turn on the pump.

ADMINISTRATION OF BLOOD PRODUCTS THROUGH A CAPPED CATHETER

Equipment

1. Blood product
2. Blood administration tubing
3. Normal saline flush bottle
4. IV administration tubing
5. Administration of 3 ml of heparinized saline in syringe with 1-inch 22-gauge needle
6. Sterile injection cap
7. Alcohol wipes
8. Sterile extension tubing
9. Stopcock

Procedure

1. Wash hands.
2. Ensure that the catheter is clamped.
3. Remove the injection cap.
4. Wipe the catheter hub with an alcohol wipe.
5. Connect extension tubing to the catheter and stopcock to the extension tubing. Connect blood administration tubing and normal saline flush tubing to stopcock. Secure all connections with tape.
6. Release the clamp and thoroughly flush the catheter with normal saline.
7. Infuse the blood product.
8. After the blood product has infused, flush the line thoroughly with normal saline.
9. Turn off the normal saline flush.
10. Clamp the catheter with the cannula clamp.
11. Disconnect the IV tubing extension from catheter.
12. Connect the injection cap to the catheter.
13. Wipe the cap with alcohol and allow it to dry.
14. Insert the needle of syringe with heparinized saline.
15. Remove the clamp.
16. Slowly inject heparinized saline.
17. Clamp the catheter while simultaneously pushing the last 0.5 ml of heparinized saline.
18. Remove the syringe.
19. Ensure that the catheter clamp is secure.

DRESSING CHANGE OF THE
HICKMAN CATHETER OR HYPERALIMENTATION
CENTRAL LINE

Because of the increased risk of infection during administration of total parenteral nutrition (TPN) the central line dressing should be changed every other day or sooner, should the dressing become soiled or loose.

Equipment

1. Two pairs of sterile gloves
2. Two packets of povidone-iodine-soaked swabs
3. Diluted hydrogen peroxide solution (half-normal saline/half-hydrogen peroxide)
4. One packet of povidone-iodine ointment
5. Five 2 × 2 gauze pads
6. Two dry swab sticks
7. Two surgical masks

Procedure

1. Wash hands.
2. Put on a mask.
3. Put a mask on the patient.
4. Place the patient in the supine position with the bed raised to a comfortable working position.
5. Have the patient turn her head to the opposite side of which you are working.
6. Put on the first pair of sterile gloves.
7. Prepare the sterile field and assemble the equipment.
8. Remove the old dressing from the patient and inspect the insertion site of the catheter for signs of infection:
   a. Redness
   b. Swelling
   c. Pain
   d. Purulent exudate
9. Remove the gloves and put on the second pair of sterile gloves.
10. Take one swab soaked with hydrogen peroxide and begin cleansing the skin. Start directly at the insertion site and clean in a circular fashion without retracing the area already done. (Do approximately a 3-inch diameter and repeat using a new swab until the area appears clean.)

11. Repeat the cleansing procedure using a povidone-iodine-soaked swab. Repeat if necessary using a new swab.
12. Allow povidone-iodine to dry for 2 minutes.
13. Place one 2 × 2 gauze pad prepared with povidone-iodine ointment over the insertion site.
14. Apply skin prep on skin around insertion site.
15. Place two 2 × 2 gauze pads to cover the catheter extending to, but not covering, the catheter hub.
16. Using 3-inch Transpore tape, apply approximately a 5.5-inch strip of tape over the gauze pads to form an occlusive seal.
17. A transparent occlusive dressing (e.g., Tegaderm) can be used in lieu of gauze and tape.

MANAGEMENT OF THE NONFUNCTIONING CATHETER

1. Fill a syringe with 3 ml of heparin 1,000 U/ml.
2. Inject the 3 ml of heparin into the catheter.
3. Place the cap on the catheter and do not disturb for 1 hour.
4. After 1 hour, using a 5-ml syringe, attempt to aspirate.
5. Irrigate with heparinized saline 5–10 ml (100 U/ml).
6. If the catheter is still blocked, repeat steps 1 and 2, clamp catheter overnight, then attempt to aspirate. If catheter still does not function, follow the streptokinase procedure.

EMERGENCY REPAIR OF THE HICKMAN CATHETER IF THE CATHETER BREAKS OR IS CUT DURING USE

1. Immediately clamp the line above the cut, close to the exit site.
2. Insert a 14-gauge Angiocath at the cut, and tape securely.
3. Place an injection cap on the Angiocath.
4. Irrigate with heparinized saline.
5. Make arrangements for permanent repair.

STREPTOKINASE FOR MANAGING THE CATHETER OCCLUDED WITH FIBRIN OR BLOOD CLOT

Equipment

1. Streptokinase 125,000 U/ml
2. Heparinized saline (100 U/ml)
3. Two to four 3-ml syringes

4. One to two 10-ml syringes
5. Cannula clamp(s)

Procedure

1. The dye study must be done before using streptokinase if the catheter is not radiopaque; this is to establish catheter position.
2. Inject 1.5 ml of streptokinase solution into the catheter(s). Both lumens of a double-lumen catheter must be treated. Clamp catheter(s) after injection, cap, and tape.
3. Catheter must be kept clamped for 6 hours minimum, preferably overnight.
4. Withdraw streptokinase from catheter(s) at the end of treatment using the 3-ml syringe(s).
5. Flush catheter(s) vigorously (after withdrawal of streptokinase) with heparinized saline (6–10 ml flush in each lumen).

Note: This procedure should be used after all other attempts at management have been tried and only after position of the catheter has been verified.

Possible Reactions to Streptokinase

1. Headache
2. Fever and chills
3. Bleeding that may be seen after repeated use.
4. Allergic reactions have been seen in 3% of treated patients.

SUGGESTED READINGS

Brincker H, Saeter G: Fifty-five patient years experience with a totally implantable system for intravenous chemotherapy. Cancer 57:1124, 1986

Brothers TE, Von Moll LK, Niederhuber JE, et al: Experience with subcutaneous infusion ports in three hundred patients. Surg Gynecol Obstet 166:295, 1988

Dardik H, Sussman BC, Kahn M, et al: Lysis of arterial clot by intravenous or intra-arterial administration of streptokinase. Surg Gynecol Obstet 158:137, 1984

Fraschini G, Jadeja J, Lawson M, et al: Local infusion of urokinase for the lysis of thrombosis associated with permanent central venous catheters in cancer patients. J Clin Oncol 5:672, 1987

Gyves JW, Eusminger WD, Niederhuber JE, et al: A totally implanted injection port system for blood sampling and chemotherapy administration. JAMA 251:2538, 1984

Lokich JJ, Bothe A Jr, Benoti P, et al: Complications and management of implanted venous access catheters. J Clin Oncol 3:710, 1985

Malviya V, Lubicz S, Deppe G, et al: Use of indwelling right atrial catheter in gynecological oncology: A preliminary report. Gynecol Oncol 17:149, 1984

Reed WP, Newman KA: An improved technique for the insertion of Hickman catheters in patients with thrombocytopenia and granulocytopenia. Surg Gynecol Obstet 156:355, 1983

Reed WP, Newman KA, de Jongh C, et al: Prolonged venous access for chemotherapy by means of the Hickman catheter. Cancer 52:185, 1983

Stanislav GV, Fitzgibbons RJ Jr, Bailey RT Jr, et al: Reliability of implantable central venous access devices in patients with cancer. Arch Surg 122:1280, 1987

Strum S, McDermed J, Korn A, et al: Improved methods for venous access: The Port-A-Cath, a totally implanted catheter system. J Clin Oncol 4:596, 1986

12

Cervical Intraepithelial Neoplasia

Cervical cytology as a screening technique for cervical cancer has had a definite impact in reducing the morbidity from this disease in the population. The colposcope is now recognized as a complement to the Papanicolaou smear. It aids the clinician in the careful inspection of the entire transformation zone, the area of change from columnar epithelium to squamous epithelium. Areas of abnormality are identified and directed biopsies obtained. The use of the colposcope in evaluating women with abnormal cervical cytology has reduced the number of cervical conizations by 80–90%. What follows are general guidelines on the evaluation and management of the patient with cervical intraepithelial neoplasia. The reader is referred to the many available colposcopy textbooks and to instructors for a more complete coverage of colposcopy. Colposcopy should be performed by physicians with formal training in this technique and who have had supervised experience.

COLPOSCOPY CANDIDATES

1. Women with a cervical lesion on inspection, with or without an abnormal cytologic diagnosis, should have a biopsy of the lesion (Fig. 12-1).
2. Women with no obvious lesion and a cytologic diagnosis of invasive cancer or cervical intraepithelial neoplasia (CIN) should undergo colposcopic evaluation.
3. Women with a cytologic diagnosis of atypical squamous cells should undergo colposcopic evaluation, since 20–30% will harbor cervical intraepithelial neoplasia.

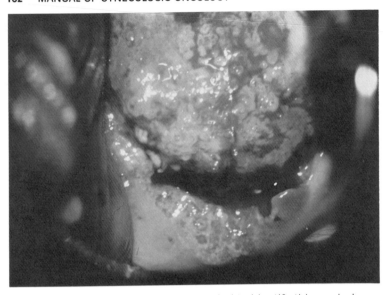

FIG. 12-1. The colposcope was not needed to identify this cervical cancer. The Papanicolaou smear was unsatisfactory due to a "dirty background," which did not allow for adequate examination of the squamous cells.

COLPOSCOPIC EVALUATION

GOALS OF THE COLPOSCOPIC EVALUATION

1. Rule out invasive cancer.
2. Localize the abnormal sites for biopsy.
3. Evaluate the extent of the lesion.
4. Identify and inspect the entire transformation zone (Fig. 12-2).

PROCEDURE

1. Gross inspection
2. Colposcopic examination of the undisturbed cervix.
3. Cervical smear obtained for cytology (Papanicolaou smear)
4. Application of 3% acetic acid
5. Colposcopic examination
   a. Starting with low magnification

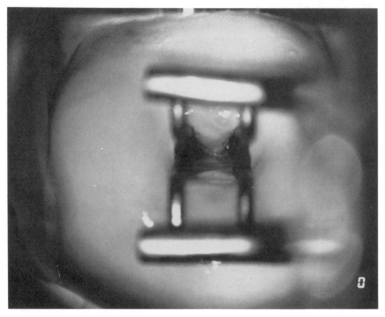

FIG. 12-2. Inspection of the transformation zone with the endocervical speculum.

    b. Green filter used to highlight vascular changes
6. Colposcopically directed punch biopsies using Kevorkian forceps or similar instrument
7. Endocervical curettage using Kevorkian curette or similar instrument.

CRITERIA OF ADEQUACY

The colposcopic examination is considered adequate if:

1. The entire transformation zone is visualized.
2. The identified lesions are seen in their entirety.
3. The area of abnormality does not occupy more than 50% of the face of the cervix.

TREATMENT GUIDELINES

1. Patients with adequate colposcopy (as defined above), with CIN 1, CIN 2, or CIN 3, and negative endocervical curettage are candidates for ablative therapy (e.g., cryosurgery, laser vaporization).
2. Patients with inadequate colposcopy or endocervical curettings with CIN require cervical conization.
3. Patients with a cytologic diagnosis of invasive cancer and whose colposcopically directed biopsies only show CIN and patients with a cytologic diagnosis of CIN 3 and whose colposcopically directed biopsies show CIN 1 require further evaluation with cervical conization.
4. Patients with a diagnosis of microinvasion on colposcopically directed biopsy require cervical conization.

TREATMENT MODALITIES

Our preferred ablative treatment modalities are laser and cryosurgery. Cure rates with these two modalities are similar (85–90%). The cryosurgery is less expensive and more convenient. Patients treated by either modality will experience a heavy malodorous discharge. The discharge lasts approximately 2 weeks with the laser as compared with 4 weeks with cryosurgery. Healing after laser therapy is more physiologic, with the transformation zone easily seen at the portio in more than 85% of patients. It has been suggested that better results are obtained when the laser, rather than cryosurgery, is used for the treatment of CIN with deep glandular involvement.

CRYOSURGERY TECHNIQUE

1. Cleansing of the cervix
2. Selection of a cryosurgery tip that will completely cover the transformation zone and the lesions
3. Application of lubricant (e.g., K-Y Jelly) to the cryosurgery tip
4. Application of the tip against the cervix; freezing for 3 minutes
5. Inspection of the iceball margins; iceball should extend 4–5 mm around the probe and beyond the lesion
6. Thawing of iceball
7. Inspection of the treated area

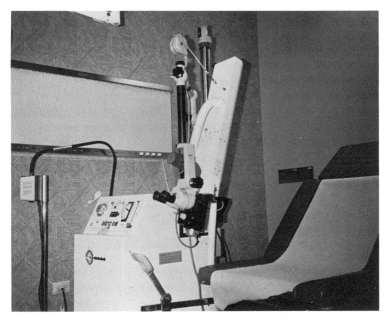

FIG. 12-3. Cavitron laser coupled to Zeiss colposcope.

8. Refreezing for 2 minutes
9. Inspection of iceball margins

LASER TECHNIQUE

The use of this modality of therapy requires formal instruction in laser biophysics, complete knowledge of the safety measures to be observed when using this form of energy, and prior supervised experience. Expertise in colposcopy is also required (Fig. 12-3).

1. Using a 2-mm spot size and a power density of approximately 800 W/cm^2, the transformation zone is outlined with a 2- to 3-mm lateral margin. This can be done by firing the laser in bursts of 500 msec or in the continuous mode if the surgeon has extensive experience.
2. The transformation zone is divided into four quadrants and vaporized one quadrant at a time.

3. The lower quadrants are vaporized first to a measured depth of 5–7 mm.
4. For vaporization, the laser beam is moved over the transformation zone in horizontal, vertical, and oblique directions.
5. After completing the vaporization, Monsel's solution is applied to the laser wound.

If the procedure is done in an office setting, a nonsteroidal antiinflammatory agent (NSAID) can be given a half-hour before the operation. A few patients will require a paracervical block.

FOLLOW-UP

1. After laser or cryosurgery, patients are asked to restrain from sexual intercourse, douching, and use of tampons for 14 days.
2. Patients are examined 4–6 weeks after the procedure to document healing and identify possible complications (e.g., infection, cervical stenosis).
3. Thereafter, patients are evaluated every 4–6 months with cervical cytology. Repeat colposcopy and directed biopsies are performed if the cytology is abnormal.
4. Follow-up with yearly Papanicolaou smears is done after 12–18 months of close follow-up without evidence of CIN persistence or recurrence.

SUGGESTED READINGS

Anderson MC, Hartley RB: Cervical crypt involvement by intraepithelial neoplasia. Obstet Gynecol 55:546, 1980

Benedet JL, Miller DM, Nickerson KG, et al: The results of cryosurgical treatment of cervical intraepithelial neoplasia at one, five, and ten years. Am J Obstet Gynecol 157:268, 1987

Bryson SCP, Leneham P, Lickrish GM: The treatment of grade 3 cervical intraepithelial neoplasia with cryotherapy: An 11 year experience. Am J Obstet Gynecol 151:201, 1985

Creasman WT, Hinshaw WA, Clarke-Pearson DL: Cryosurgery in the management of cervical intraepithelial neoplasia. Obstet Gynecol 63:145, 1984

Davis GL, Hernandez E, Davis JL, et al: Atypical squamous cells in Papanicolaou smears. Obstet Gynecol 69:43, 1987

Ferenczy A: Comparison of cryo- and carbon dioxide laser therapy for cervical intraepithelial neoplasia. Obstet Gynecol 66:793, 1985

Giuntoli RL, Atkinson BF, Ernst CS, et al: Atkinson's Correlative Atlas of Colposcopy, Cytology and Histopathology. 1st Ed. JB Lippincott, Philadelphia, 1987

Grainger DA, Roberts DK, Wells MM, et al: The value of endocervical curettage in the management of the patient with abnormal cervical cytologic findings. Am J Obstet Gynecol 156:625, 1987

Jones DED, Creasman WT, Dombroski, RA, et al: Evaluation of the atypical Pap smear. Am J Obstet Gynecol 157:544, 1987

Noumoff JS: Atypia in cervical cytology as a risk factor for intraepithelial neoplasia. Am J Obstet Gynecol 156:628, 1987

Reiter RC: Management of initial atypical cytology: A randomized prospective study. Obstet Gynecol 68:237, 1986

Ridgley R, Hernandez E, Cruz C, et al: Abnormal Papanicolaou smears after earlier smears with atypical squamous cells. J Reprod Med 33:285, 1988

Stenkvist B, Bergstrom R, Eklund G, et al: Papanicolaou smear screening and cervical cancer: What can you expect? JAMA 252:1423, 1984

Stever MR, Hernandez E, Miyazawa K: Laser vaporization for the treatment of cervical intraepithelial neoplasia in a teaching hospital. Journal American Osteopathic Association 88:1269, 1988

Townsend DE, Richart RM: Cryotherapy and carbon dioxide laser managment of cervical intraepithelial neoplasia: A controlled comparison. Obstet Gynecol 61:75, 1983

Wetrich DW: An analysis of the factors involved in the colposcopic evaluation of 2194 patients with abnormal Papanicolaou smears. Am J Obstet Gynecol 154:1339, 1986

Appendix I

Bowel Preparation Prior to Radical Pelvic Surgery, Intestinal Surgery, Gynecologic Surgery Requiring Intestinal Preparation, Sigmoidoscopy, or Colonoscopy

1. The patient requiring bowel preparation for major gynecologic surgery is given a clear liquid diet for the 3 days before the scheduled surgery.
2. On preoperative days 3 and 2, the patient takes two Dulcolax tablets orally (PO).
3. On preoperative day 2, order 4 L of colonoscopy lavage solution to the ward (GoLYTELY: 125 mEq/L sodium, 10 mEq/L potassium, 80 mEq/L sulfate, 20 mEq/L bicarbonate, 35 mEq/L chloride, 80 mEq/L polyethylene glycol). Keep refrigerated.
4. Obtain weight, serum electrolytes, and complete blood count (CBC) before initiating the GoLYTELY.
5. The patient takes 1 L/hr of GoLYTELY early on preoperative day 1 until the rectal effluent is clear. (GoLYTELY tastes like salted soapy water, keep ice cold.)
6. Give Reglan 10 mg intramuscularly (IM) 1 hour before the patient starts taking the GoLYTELY.
7. Give Erythromycin Base Filmtab 1 g and Neomycin 1 g PO at 1300, 1400, and 2300 hours.
8. The evening before surgery, the patient receives soap sud enemas until clear.
9. Obtain weight and serum electrolytes after completing the intestinal preparation.
10. Some patients (e.g., sigmoidoscopy, colonoscopy, pelvic masses) will only need a 1-day bowel prep (e.g., GoLYTELY only).

SUGGESTED READINGS

Davis GR, Santa Ana CA, Morawski SG, et al: Development of a lavage solution associated with minimal water and electrolyte absorption or secretion. Gastroenterology 78:991, 1980

Thomas G, Brozinsky S, Isenberg JI, et al: Patient acceptance and effectiveness of a balanced lavage solution (Golytely) versus the standard preparation for colonoscopy. Gastroenterology 82:435, 1982

Appendix II

Staging of Gynecologic Malignancies According to the International Federation of Gynecology and Obstetrics (FIGO) Classification*

I. ENDOMETRIUM

Stage 0   Carcinoma in situ. Histologic findings suspicious of malignancy. Cases of stage 0 should not be included in any therapeutic statistics.

Stage I   The carcinoma is confined in the corpus.
Stage IA   The length of the uterine cavity is 8 cm or less.
Stage IB   The length of the uterine cavity is greater than 8 cm.
Stage I cases should be subgrouped according to the histologic degree of differentiation:

      G1   Highly differentiated glandular carcinoma.
      G2   Differentiated glandular carcinoma with partly solid areas.
      G3   Predominantly solid or entirely undifferentiated carcinomas.

Stage II   The carcinoma involves the corpus and cervix.

Stage III   The carcinoma has extended outside the uterus, but not outside the true pelvis.

Stage IV   The carcinoma has extended outside the true pelvis or has obviously involved the mucosa of the bladder or rectum. Bullous edema, as such, does not permit allotment of a case to stage IV.

---

* Sections I through V are adapted from the classification accepted by FIGO on April 12, 1970 and September 1985. From Acta Obstet Gynecol Scand 50:1, 1971 and Gynecol Oncol 25:383, 1986, with permission.

II. CERVIX

Stage 0   Carcinoma in situ. Cases of stage 0 should not be included in any therapeutic statistics.

Stage I   The carcinoma is strictly confined to the cervix (extension to the corpus should be disregarded).

Stage IA   Preclinical carcinomas of the cervix, that is, those diagnosed only by microscopy.

Stage IA1   Minimal microscopically evident stromal invasion.

Stage IA2   Lesions detected microscopically that can be measured. The upper limit of the measurement should not show a depth of invasion of more than 5 mm taken from the base of the epithelium, either surface or glandular, from which it originates, and a second dimension, the horizontal spread, must not exceed 7 mm. Larger lesions should be staged as IB.

Stage IB   Lesions of greater dimensions than stage IA2 whether seen clinically or not. Preformed space involvement should not alter the staging but should be specifically recorded so as to determine whether it should affect treatment decisions in the future.

Stage II   The carcinoma extends beyond the cervix but has not extended onto the pelvic wall; it involves the vagina, but not the lower third.

Stage IIA   No obvious parametrial involvement.

Stage IIB   Obvious parametrial involvement.

Stage III   The carcinoma has extended on to the pelvic wall. On rectal examination, there is no cancer free space between the tumor and the pelvic wall. The tumor involves the lower third of the vagina. All cases with hydronephrosis or nonfunctioning kidney that are secondary to the cancer.

Stage IIIA   Involvement of lower third of the vagina. No extension onto the pelvic wall.

Stage IIIB   Extension onto pelvic wall and/or hydronephrosis or nonfunctioning kidney.

Stage IV   The carcinoma has extended beyond the true pelvis or has clinically involved the mucosa of the bladder or rectum. Bullous edema as such does not permit a case to be allotted to stage IV.

Stage IVA   Spread of the growth to the adjacent organs.

Stage IVB   Spread to distant organs.

III. OVARY

Stage I   Growth limited to the ovaries.

Stage IA   Growth limited to one ovary; no ascites. No tumor on the external surface; capsule intact.

Stage IB   Growth limited to both ovaries; no ascites. No tumor on the external surfaces; capsule intact.

Stage IC   Tumor either stage IA or IB but with tumor on surface of one or both ovaries; or with capsule ruptured; or with ascites present containing malignant cells or with positive peritoneal washings.

Stage II   Growth involving one or both ovaries with pelvic extension.

Stage IIA   Extension and/or metastases to the uterus and/or tubes.

Stage IIB   Extension to other pelvic tissues.

Stage IIC   Tumor either stage IIA or IIB, but with tumor on surface of one or both ovaries; or with capsule(s) ruptured; or with ascites present containing malignant cells or with positive peritoneal washings.

Stage III   Tumor involving one or both ovaries with peritoneal implants outside the pelvis and/or positive retroperitoneal or inguinal nodes. Superficial liver metastasis equals stage III. Tumor is limited to the true pelvis but with histologically proven malignant extension to small bowel or omentum.

Stage IIIA   Tumor grossly limited to the true pelvis with negative nodes but with histologically confirmed microscopic seeding of abdominal peritoneal surfaces.

Stage IIIB   Tumor of one or both ovaries with histologically confirmed implants of abdominal peritoneal surfaces none exceeding 2 cm in diameter; nodes are negative.

Stage IIIC   Abdominal implants greater than 2 cm in diameter and/or positive retroperitoneal or inguinal nodes.

Stage IV   Growth involving one or both ovaries with distant metastases. If pleural effusion is present there must be positive cytology to allot a case to stage IV. Parenchymal liver metastasis equals stage IV.

IV. VAGINA

Stage 0   Carcinoma in situ.

Stage I   The carcinoma is limited to the vaginal wall.

Stage II   The carcinoma has involved the subvaginal tissue but has not extended onto the pelvic wall.

Stage III   The carcinoma has extended onto the pelvic wall.

Stage IV   The carcinoma has extended beyond the true pelvis or has involved the mucosa of the bladder or rectum. Bullous edema as such does not permit a case to be allotted to stage IV.

State IVA   Spread of the growth to adjacent organs.
Stage IVB   Spread to distant organs.

V. VULVA

Stage 0   Carcinoma in situ.

Stage I   Tumor confined to vulva—2 cm or less in diameter. Nodes are not palpable or if palpable in either groin, are mobile, not enlarged (not clinically suspicious of neoplasm).

Stage II   Tumor confined to the vulva—more than 2 cm in diameter. Nodes are not palpable or if palpable in either groin, are mobile, not enlarged (not clinically suspicious of neoplasm).

Stage III   Tumor of any size with (1) adjacent spread to the urethra, vagina, perineum, and anus, and/or (2) suspicious nodes palpable in either or both groins (enlarged, firm, and mobile, not fixed but clinically suspicious of neoplasm).

Stage IV   Tumor of any size (1) infiltrating the upper part of the urethral mucosa, bladder mucosa and/or rectal mucosa; or (2) fixed to the bone; fixed or ulcerated nodes in either or both groins. Palpable deep pelvic metastases. Distant metastases.

In addition, the following statement has been made by the International Society for the Study of Vulvar Disease:

1. That the term microinvasive cancer of the vulva be discontinued.
2. That the designation stage IA cancer of the vulva be used for a small group of lesions of the vulva and that for the purposes of study these lesions be solitary and confined to a maximum of 2 cm in diameter and 1-mm depth of stromal invasion.

VI. FALLOPIAN TUBE

The International Federation of Gynecology and Obstetrics does not have a classification for fallopian tube cancer. The following classification proposed by Dodson et al. is widely used.*

Stage I	Growth limited to the tube.
Stage IA	Growth limited to one tube.
Stage IB	Growth limited to both tubes.
Stage IC	Tumor either stage IA or IB but with ascites or positive peritoneal washings.
Stage II	Growth involving one or both tubes with pelvic extension.
Stage IIA	Extension and/or metastases to the uterus and/or ovaries.
Stage IIB	Extension to other pelvic tissues.
Stage IIC	Tumor either stage IIA or IIB but with ascites or positive peritoneal washings.
Stage III	Growth involving one or both tubes with intraperitoneal metastases outside the pelvis and/or positive retroperitoneal nodes.
Stage IV	Growth involving one or both tubes with distant metastases; if pleural effusion present, must have positive cytology; parenchymal liver metastases equal stage IV.

* Staging classification from Maxson WZ, Stehman FB, Ulbright TM, et al: Primary carcinoma of the fallopian tube: Evidence for activity of cisplatin combination therapy. Gynecol Oncol 26:305, 1987, as modified from Dodson MG, Ford, Jr, JH, Averette HE: Clinical aspects of fallopian tube carcinoma. Obstet Gynecol 36:935, 1970, with permission.

Index

Page numbers followed by *f* indicate figures; page numbers followed by *t* indicate tables.